Burn Rehabilitation

Guest Editors

PETER C. ESSELMAN, MD
KAREN J. KOWALSKE, MD

PHYSICAL MEDICINE AND REHABILITATION CLINICS OF NORTH AMERICA

www.pmr.theclinics.com

Consulting Editor
GEORGE H. KRAFT, MD, MS

May 2011 • Volume 22 • Number 2

SAUNDERS an imprint of ELSEVIER, Inc.

W.B. SAUNDERS COMPANY
A Division of Elsevier Inc.

1600 John F. Kennedy Boulevard • Suite 1800 • Philadelphia, Pennsylvania 19103

http://www.theclinics.com

PHYSICAL MEDICINE AND REHABILITATION CLINICS OF NORTH AMERICA Volume 22, Number 2
May 2011 ISSN 1047-9651, ISBN-13: 978-1-4557-0491-0

Editor: Debora Dellapena
Developmental Editor: Donald Mumford

Photocopying
Single photocopies of single articles may be made for personal use as allowed by national copyright laws. Permission of the Publisher and payment of a fee is required for all other photocopying, including multiple or systematic copying, copying for advertising or promotional purposes, resale, and all forms of document delivery. Special rates are available for educational institutions that wish to make photocopies for non-profit educational classroom use. For information on how to seek permission visit www.elsevier.com/permissions or call: (+44) 1865 843830 (UK)/(+1) 215 239 3804 (USA).

Derivative Works
Subscribers may reproduce tables of contents or prepare lists of articles including abstracts for internal circulation within their institutions. Permission of the Publisher is required for resale or distribution outside the institution. Permission of the Publisher is required for all other derivative works, including compilations and translations (please consult www.elsevier.com/permissions).

Electronic Storage or Usage
Permission of the Publisher is required to store or use electronically any material contained in this journal, including any article or part of an article (please consult www.elsevier.com/permissions). Except as outlined above, no part of this publication may be reproduced, stored in a retrieval system or transmitted in any form or by any means, electronic, mechanical, photocopying, recording or otherwise, without prior written permission of the Publisher.

Notice
No responsibility is assumed by the Publisher for any injury and/or damage to persons or property as a matter of products liability, negligence or otherwise, or from any use or operation of any methods, products, instructions or ideas contained in the material herein. Because of rapid advances in the medical sciences, in particular, independent verification of diagnoses and drug dosages should be made.

Although all advertising material is expected to conform to ethical (medical) standards, inclusion in this publication does not constitute a guarantee or endorsement of the quality or value of such product or of the claims made of it by its manufacturer.

Reprints. For copies of 100 or more of articles in this publication, please contact the Commercial Reprints Department, Elsevier Inc., 360 Park Avenue South, New York, NY 10010-1710. Tel.: 212-633-3812; Fax: 212-462-1935; E-mail: reprints@elsevier.com.

Physical Medicine and Rehabilitation Clinics of North America (ISSN 1047-9651) is published quarterly by Elsevier Inc., 360 Park Avenue South, New York, NY 10010-1710. Months of issue are February, May, August, and November. Business and Editorial Offices: 1600 John F. Kennedy Blvd., Suite 1800, Philadelphia, PA 19103-2899. Customer Service Office: 3251 Riverport Lane, Maryland Heights, MO 63043. Periodicals postage paid at New York, NY and additional mailing offices. Subscription price per year is $230.00 (US individuals), $414.00 (US institutions), $122.00 (US students), $280.00 (Canadian individuals), $540.00 (Canadian institutions), $175.00 (Canadian students), $345.00 (foreign individuals), $540.00 (foreign institutions), and $175.00 (foreign students). Foreign air speed delivery is included in all *Clinics* subscription prices. All prices are subject to change without notice. **POSTMASTER:** Send address changes to *Physical Medicine and Rehabilitation Clinics of North America*, Customer Service Office: Elsevier Health Sciences Division, Subscription Customer Service, 3251 Riverport Lane, Maryland Heights, MO 63043. **Customer Service: 1-800-654-2452 (US). From outside of the United States, call 314-447-8871. Fax: 314-447-8029. E-mail: JournalsCustomer Service-usa@elsevier.com (for print support); JournalsOnlineSupport-usa@elsevier.com (for online support).**

Physical Medicine and Rehabilitation Clinics of North America is indexed in *Excerpta Medica, MEDLINE/ PubMed (Index Medicus), Cinahl,* and *Cumulative Index to Nursing and Allied Health Literature.*

Printed and bound by CPI Group (UK) Ltd, Croydon, CR0 4YY

Transferred to Digital Print 2011

Contributors

CONSULTING EDITOR

GEORGE H. KRAFT, MD
Alvord Professor of Multiple Sclerosis Research; Professor, Department of Rehabilitation Medicine and Adjunct Professor, Department of Neurology, University of Washington, Seattle, Washington

GUEST EDITORS

PETER C. ESSELMAN, MD
Professor and Chair, Department of Rehabilitation Medicine, University of Washington Burn Center, Harborview Medical Center, Seattle, Washington

KAREN J. KOWALSKE, MD
Professor and Chair, Department of Physical Medicine and Rehabilitation, University of Texas Southwestern Medical Center, Dallas, Texas

AUTHORS

BRETT D. ARNOLDO, MD
Associate Professor of Surgery, Division Burns/Trauma/Critical Care, Department of Surgery; Co-Director, Burn Center, Parkland Memorial Hospital, University of Texas Southwestern Medical Center, Dallas, Texas

RYAN BLANCK, BS, CPO
Upper Extremity Prosthetics Specialist, Department of Orthopedics and Rehabilitation, Brooke Army Medical Center, Center for the Intrepid, Fort Sam Houston, Texas

BARBARA J. DE LATEUR, MD, MS
Distinguished Service Professor; Lawrence Cardinal Shehan Professor and Director Emerita, Department of Physical Medicine and Rehabilitation, The Johns Hopkins University, Johns Hopkins Medical Institutions, Baltimore, Maryland

WILLIAM S. DEWEY, PT
Program Manager, United States Army Burn Center Rehabilitation Department, United States Army Institute of Surgical Research, Fort Sam Houston, San Antonio, Texas

PETER C. ESSELMAN, MD
Professor and Chair, Department of Rehabilitation Medicine, University of Washington Burn Center, Harborview Medical Center, Seattle, Washington

JOHN R. FERGASON, BA, CPO
Chief Prosthetist, Department of Orthopedics and Rehabilitation, Brooke Army Medical Center, Center for the Intrepid, Fort Sam Houston, San Antonio, Texas

VINCENT GABRIEL, MD, MSc, FRCPC
Director, Burn Rehabilitation, Fire Fighters Burn Treatment Centre, Foothills Medical Centre; Assistant Professor, Division of Physical Medicine and Rehabilitation, Department of Clinical Neurosciences, University of Calgary, Calgary, Alberta, Canada

JOHN L. HUNT, MD
Professor of Surgery, Division Burns/Trauma/Critical Care, Department of Surgery; Attending Surgeon, Parkland Memorial Hospital, University of Texas Southwestern Medical Center, Dallas, Texas

MATTHEW B. KLEIN, MD, MS, FACS
David and Nancy Auth-Washington Research Foundation Endowed Chair for Restorative Burn Surgery, Division of Plastic Surgery, Harborview Medical Center, University of Washington Regional Burn Center, Seattle, Washington

KAREN J. KOWALSKE, MD
Professor and Chair, Department of Physical Medicine and Rehabilitation, University of Texas Southwestern Medical Center, Dallas, Texas

INGRID S. PARRY, MS, PT
Rehabilitation Research Therapist, Shriners Hospital for Children, Northern California, Sacramento, California

†GARY F. PURDUE, MD
Professor of Surgery, Division Burns/Trauma/Critical Care, Department of Surgery; Co-Director, Burn Center, Parkland Memorial Hospital, University of Texas Southwestern Medical Center, Dallas, Texas

HUAGUANG DAVID QU, MD, MS
Department of Physical Medicine and Rehabilitation, Harvard Medical School, Boston, Massachusetts

REG L. RICHARD, MS, PT
Clinical Research Coordinator, Burn Rehabilitation, United States Army Institute of Surgical Research, Fort Sam Houston, San Antonio, Texas

JEFFERY C. SCHNEIDER, MD
Medical Director, Trauma, Burn and Orthopedic Program; Assistant Professor, Department of Physical Medicine and Rehabilitation, Harvard Medical School, Spaulding Rehabilitation Hospital, Boston, Massachusetts

WENDY S. SHORE, PhD
Research Associate, Department of Physical Medicine and Rehabilitation, The Johns Hopkins University, Johns Hopkins Medical Institutions, Baltimore, Maryland

SHELLEY A. WIECHMAN, PhD
Associate Professor, Department of Rehabilitation Medicine, University of Washington School of Medicine, Seattle, Washington

†Deceased.

Contents

Burns are ubiquitous injuries in modern society, with virtually all adults having sustained a burn at some point in their lives. The skin is the largest organ of the body, basically functioning to protect self from non-self. Burn injury to the skin is painful, resource-intensive, and often associated with scarring, contracture formation, and long-term disability. Larger burns are associated with morbidity and mortality disproportionate to their initial appearance. Electrical and chemical burns are less common injuries but are often associated with significant morbidity.

The goals of burn wound care are removal of nonviable tissue, prevention of infection, and facilitation of wound healing, while controlling pain and maximizing outcome. This article reviews the basic pathophysiology of burn wounds; describes the evaluation of the depth, location, and extent of the wound; and discusses the myriad of wound care products on the market including their strengths and weaknesses. This article guides the reader through wound assessment and designing the appropriate treatment plan.

Whether a patient with burn injury is an adult or child, contracture management should be the primary focus of burn rehabilitation throughout the continuum of care. Positioning and splinting are crucial components of a comprehensive burn rehabilitation program that emphasizes contracture prevention. The emphasis of these devices throughout the phases of rehabilitation fluctuates to meet the changing needs of patients with burn injury. Early, effective, and consistent use of positioning devices and splints is recommended for successful management of burn scar contracture.

the emphasis on burn reconstruction. There are an increasing number of persons surviving extensive injury who may have long-term reconstructive needs. Burn reconstruction, just as acute burn care, requires a coordinated team approach from initial consultation through recovery and rehabilitation. Clearly, in the future, one can expect evolution in surgical techniques and technologies that can improve the function and appearance of persons with burn injury.

THE CLINICS ARE NOW AVAILABLE ONLINE!

Access your subscription at:
www.theclinics.com

Dedication

Gary Purdue

August 19, 1945–October 3, 2010

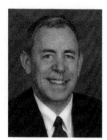

Gary Purdue, MD

"Well done, good and faithful servant."

This issue is dedicated to the memory of our friend and colleague, Dr Gary Purdue. A native of Elmira, New York, Dr Purdue received his medical degree from Jefferson Medical College in Pennsylvania in 1976 and in 1981 completed his general surgery residency at Mercy Hospital in Pittsburgh. Just before Gary entered medical school, his father was electrocuted in a boating accident, which reinforced his desire to become a physician and channeled his energies toward burn care. He served as the co-director of the Parkland Health and Hospital Systems burn unit for 22 years. Parkland has one of the largest burn units in the nation, treating almost 1,000 burn victims annually. He was a professor and chief of the burn division of the department of surgery at the University of Texas Southwestern Medical Center, where he was a valued faculty member for nearly 30 years. He was a past president of the American Burn Association and an international leader in burn care. Gary's career was marked by outstanding clinical skills, cutting-edge research, and hands-on teaching and mentoring skills.

Gary Purdue can best be described as a man of passion. He was passionate about his family, passionate about his profession, passionate about his faith, and passionate about his relationships with others. He was a crusader for the victim and yet compassionate to all. Gary laughed loudly, loved fiercely, and lived a life of the highest integrity.

He had a number of "proverbs" that all in his lineage continue to use daily:

"It is better to be better and not know why than to know why and not be better."

For operating on geriatric patients, "you can easily rob the bank once and get away with it but the second time the guard is waiting for you."

On how much lotion to apply, "your skin should be as greasy as the edge of your nose at the end of the day."

He was and is, in many ways, still a role model and mentor to us all. He will be sorely missed and lovingly remembered by the burn community.

Phys Med Rehabil Clin N Am 22 (2011) ix
doi:10.1016/j.pmr.2011.03.005
1047-9651/11/$ – see front matter © 2011 Elsevier Inc. All rights reserved.

Foreword

Burn Rehabilitation

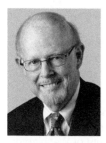

George H. Kraft, MD
Consulting Editor

As you will have noted upon opening this issue, it begins with a dedication to the memory of Gary F. Purdue, an article author who died a few months before publication. His passing is noted with sadness.

This issue of the *Physical Medicine and Rehabilitation Clinics of North America* is the first where our two guest editors are department chairs.

I would like to thank Dr Peter Esselman, Chair of the Department of Rehabilitation Medicine at the University of Washington, and Dr Karen Kowalske, Chair at the University of Texas, Dallas for taking on this important topic and bringing it to fruition. The topic, too, is the first on Burn Rehabilitation in the long history of this series.

Burn rehabilitation is not the most commonly encountered problem seen by physiatrists, which is exactly why it is being presented in the *Clinics*—the most retrievable source of medical information for physiatrists. This series is a "living textbook" and can be kept on the physician's office shelf, just like any other text. But the advantage is that as a new topic comes out (such as the topic being reviewed in this issue) or new information on previously published topics becomes available, they can be published quickly and sent to the reader. The whole series provides an important and easily retrievable source of medical information for the practitioner.

When the practicing physician is consulted and asked to participate in the care of a burn patient, he/she will now be able to pull this issue from the shelf and review the pertinent sections. Or, if a PubMed search is made, relevant *Clinics* articles will show up.

The article by Drs Purdue, Amoldo, and Hunt on assessment and management of burns leads off this issue, followed by an article by Dr Kowalske on the care of burn wounds. Next, contributors Dewey, Richard, and Parry explain positioning, splinting, and contracture management.

After this, Dr Kowalske writes about hand burns, and Drs Schneider and Qu discuss neurologic and musculoskeletal complications of burns. Fergason and Blanck have written an article on prosthetic management of the burn amputation, and Gabriel

Phys Med Rehabil Clin N Am 22 (2011) xi–xii
doi:10.1016/j.pmr.2011.03.006

explains management of the hypertrophic scar. Next, Dr Klein has an article about burn reconstruction.

Moving into the important area of a burn's psycho-social impact, Weichman has written an article on management of psychosocial issues, as well as pain and itch after burn injuries. Drs deLateur and Shore discuss the role of post-burn exercise. The issue concludes with an article on community integration after burn injury by Dr Esselman.

As noted, this is the first issue in this series on the role of rehabilitation in the management of burns. Concepts and techniques are presented. I am confident that when a physiatrist is asked to participate in the care of a patient with burns, this issue of the *Clinics* will serve as an invaluable resource.

George H. Kraft, MD
Department of Rehabilitation Medicine
University of Washington
1959 NE Pacific Street, RJ-30
Seattle, WA 98195, USA

E-mail address:
ghkraft@uw.edu

Preface

Burn Rehabilitation

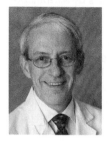 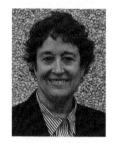

Peter C. Esselman, MD   Karen J. Kowalske, MD
Guest Editors

This edition of *Physical Medicine and Rehabilitation Clinics of North America* reviews the acute management of burn injuries and the most frequent consequences of burn injuries including hypertrophic scarring, amputations, neuromuscular problems, and management of contractures, pain, itch, and psychosocial issues. Treatment options such as splinting, positioning, exercise, and surgical reconstruction are covered as well as community integration. The optimal treatment of burn injuries is provided by a coordinated interdisciplinary team that is aware of long-term rehabilitation issues during the acute management of burn injuries and provides long-term comprehensive rehabilitation. The ultimate goal for the individual with a burn injury is to maximize function and return to previous activities with an optimal quality of life.

The incidence of burn injuries has decreased over time with improved safety measures such as smoke alarms and workplace safety. The American Burn Association reports that in the United States there are 500,000 individuals every year receiving medical treatment for burn injuries. There are 3,500 deaths per year and 45,000 individuals are hospitalized every year. Of those hospitalized, 25,000 are admitted to hospitals with burn centers. They report the cause of burn injuries in those admitted to burn centers to be fire/flame (42%), scald injury (31%), contact with a hot object (9%), chemical (3%), electrical (4%), and other causes (11%). In 66% of cases the injury occurred at home, 10% at the workplace, 8% on the street/highway, and 16% in other location. Like many traumatic injuries, burn injuries in the United States occur predominantly in men (70%) compared to women (30%). Mortality has also decreased over time, with 94.8% survival in individuals admitted to burn centers.[1]

Survival of large burns has greatly improved with advances in resuscitation, early excision and grafting, and infection control measures. The risk of mortality increases

Phys Med Rehabil Clin N Am 22 (2011) xiii–xv
doi:10.1016/j.pmr.2011.03.002
1047-9651/11/$ – see front matter © 2011 Elsevier Inc. All rights reserved.

pmr.theclinics.com

with the size of the burn, with the presence of inhalation injury, and in the elderly. In the 1980s, a burn that involved 60% to 70% Total Body Surface Area (TBSA) was often fatal and now patients are routinely surviving 80% to 90% TBSA burn injuries. Survival and outcome have improved with the establishment of organized burn centers and almost all individuals (96%) in the United States live within two hours by air transport of a burn center.[2] Increased survival of large burn injuries has emphasized the need for treatment teams with a focus on comprehensive rehabilitation. Individuals with large burn injuries often have severe contractures, joint deformities, amputations, psychosocial issues, and other complications addressed by the rehabilitation team.

The rehabilitation management of individuals with burn injuries involves prolonged and focused intervention at different levels of care. In many traumatic injuries, there is often a period of time focused on acute care/surgical treatment followed by a focus on rehabilitation, but the ideal treatment of an individual with a burn injury includes rehabilitation as part of the acute management and long-term rehabilitation coordinated with surgical reconstruction. A 2008 article by Richard and coauthors discussed the continuum of rehabilitation care of burn injuries.[3] The authors describe an early rehabilitation phase starting at the time of admission to the burn unit and continuing until the patient's wounds are 50% closed or skin grafting has begun. This is a period of time in which rehabilitation has a focus on proper positioning, splinting, range of motion, and mobilization that will prevent long-term complications. The next phase, the intermediate phase, is during wound closure up to complete wound closure. In this phase, the rehabilitation team is more involved but works closely with the acute care team to promote wound healing while focusing on positioning and functional mobility and preventing contractures. The long-term phase is the rehabilitation intensive phase leading up to discharge from the acute care hospital and admission to inpatient rehabilitation or transition to an outpatient rehabilitation program. In this phase the primary focus is on maximizing function with therapy intervention or reconstructive surgery. During all these phases, it is important to consider psychological rehabilitation in addition to physical rehabilitation. Many patients have issues with anxiety, posttraumatic stress, depression, and body image concerns that benefit from psychological intervention.

The treatment of individuals with burn injuries present the rehabilitation treatment team with multiple unique challenges not seen in other areas of rehabilitation medicine. These often include a combination of scarring, contractures, joint deformities, weakness, and amputations along with the psychological consequences of severe burn injuries. For optimal outcomes, it is important for patients to have a coordinated rehabilitation treatment plan that includes access to psychological services and to have access to vocational rehabilitation to promote return to previous activities, including the return to work.

Peter C. Esselman, MD
Department of Rehabilitation Medicine
University of Washington Burn Center
Harborview Medical Center
University of Washington
325 9th Avenue, Box 359612
Seattle, WA 98104, USA

E-mail address:
esselman@u.washington.edu

Karen J. Kowalske, MD
Department of Physical Medicine
and Rehabilitation
University Texas SW Medical Center
5323 Harry Hines Boulevard
Dallas, TX 75390-9055, USA

E-mail address:
karen.kowalske@utsouthwestern.edu

REFERENCES

1. Burn Incidence and Treatment in the US: 2011 Fact sheet. Available at: http://www. ameriburn.org/resources_factsheet.php. Accessed March 1, 2011.
2. Klein MB, Kramer CB, Nelson J, et al. Geographic access to burn center hospitals. JAMA 2009;302(16):1774–81.
3. Richard RL, Hedman TL, Quick CD, et al. A clarion to recommit and reaffirm burn rehabilitation. J Burn Care Res 2008;29:425–32.

Acute Assessment and Management of Burn Injuries

Gary F. Purdue, MD[a,†], Brett D. Arnoldo, MD[a],*, John L. Hunt, MD[b]

KEYWORDS
• Burn • Early care • Assessment

Burns are ubiquitous injuries in modern society, with virtually all adults having sustained a burn at some point in their lives. The skin is the largest organ of the body, basically functioning to protect self from non-self. Burn injury to the skin is painful, resource-intensive, and often associated with scarring, contracture formation, and long-term disability. Larger burns are associated with morbidity and mortality disproportionate to their initial appearance. Accurate assessment of the burn patient and appropriate institution of early care are critical to optimal outcomes. Initial evaluation uses the "ABC" precepts of the Advanced Trauma Life Support (ATLS) course: airway, breathing, and circulation.[1] Additional burn-specific care is noted in the Advanced Burn Life Support (ABLS) course.[2]

Nearly all burns are completely preventable, requiring conscious thought to occur. Approximately one-third of patients admitted to burn centers are children. Most pediatric injuries are scald burns and are related to cooking, with hot beverages, soups, and microwaved foods frequent offenders. Keeping children out of the kitchen during cooking would minimize these burns. Tap water burns in both young and elderly individuals are caused by the temperature of the water heater being set too high (>120°F), and can be completely avoided by simply resetting the water heater's thermostat. Inappropriate use of highly flammable liquids, such as gasoline and lighter fluid, is a significant cause of burn injury in adults. Smoking, intoxication, suicide attempts, and assaults provide continuing sources of burn injury. Electrical and chemical burns are primarily adult injuries.

The authors have nothing to disclose.
† Deceased.
a Division Burns/Trauma/Critical Care, Department of Surgery, Burn Center, Parkland Memorial Hospital, University of Texas SW Medical Center, 5323 Harry Hines Boulevard, Dallas, TX 75390-9158, USA
b Division Burns/Trauma/Critical Care, Department of Surgery, Parkland Memorial Hospital, University of Texas SW Medical Center, 5323 Harry Hines Boulevard, Dallas, TX 75390-9158, USA
* Corresponding author.
E-mail address: brett.arnoldo@utsouthwestern.edu

Phys Med Rehabil Clin N Am 22 (2011) 201–212
doi:10.1016/j.pmr.2011.01.004
1047-9651/11/$ – see front matter © 2011 Elsevier Inc. All rights reserved.
pmr.theclinics.com

DETERMINANTS OF SEVERITY

Although burn size and depth are obvious factors in determining burn severity, the location (body part) of the burn, age of the patient, preexisting disease, and presence of trauma, including an inhalation injury, may complicate treatment.

Burns to the head and neck, hands, feet, and perineum and genitalia confer significant morbidity and mortality to the injury disproportionate to burn size. The airway originates and passes through the head and neck, requiring continual vigilance and need for airway protection, in addition to the obvious changes in appearance engendered by these burns. Hand burns require significant available skin grafts, operating time, and therapy resources disproportionate to their relatively small size. Because of the proximity of tendons and joints to the skin surface, injury is common in these structures, which are critical for normal function. Foot burns render patients immobile, and grafts in these areas are at risk for wear and tear from footwear. The perineum and genitalia are areas that are at risk for infection during burn treatment, and are also nearly impossible to immobilize for adequate graft take.

Patients younger than 2 years or older than 50 years are at higher risk of complications and death than the remaining population. In babies, thin skin, limited reserves, and high surface area–to–mass ratios contribute to this risk, whereas thinning skin and medical problems commonly associated with aging are major factors in older individuals. Young children are also at risk for burns caused by abuse. These injuries are most often scald burns from tap water, and are deeper than those seen in the general pediatric burn population and commonly involve the lower extremities, buttocks, and genitalia. Bathroom training and soiling are frequently involved as precipitating factors. Fortunately, these burns often have characteristic patterns of injury, aiding in appropriate diagnosis.[3]

Burns are not evenly distributed throughout the general population. Groups with higher-than-expected frequency of injury include the ill and disabled. These especially include the neurologically impaired, at risk for both occurrence and extreme depth. Seizures, paraplegia, and quadriplegia place these patients at special danger for both contact and scald burns. Diabetes mellitus, which makes medical care more difficult because of glycemic control, is also a risk factor for burn injury. Neuropathic pain relief through hot soaks or neuropathy insensate to heat cause patients to sustain burns from soaking or from walking on hot surfaces with inadequate foot protection. Associated chronic obstructive pulmonary disease and cardiovascular disease adversely affect outcomes. Smoking while on medically prescribed home oxygen creates a unique flash burn with minimal deep injury.

Traumatic injuries occur in addition to the burn in 5% to 15% of admitted patients. The most common causes are motor vehicle accidents, explosions, and falls sustained while escaping from the burn site. Evaluation and treatment of traumatic injuries takes precedence over treatment of the burn, with the caveat that maintenance of body temperature, airway protection, and appropriate burn fluid resuscitation must be achieved.

Burn Depth

Burn depth is a product of temperature, duration of exposure, and skin thickness, with depth being described in degrees based on its relationship to total skin thickness. Most burns have areas that are of mixed depth, with deeper burns often occurring in areas of thinner skin thickness.

First-degree burns involve only the epidermis or topmost layer of skin. They are recognized by their erythematous appearance and lack of blisters or skin separation.

When rubbed with the gloved finger, the burn tissue does not separate from the underlying dermis (ie, negative Nikolsky's sign). Although more commonly used for dermatologic diseases, Nikolsky's sign is also a reliable differentiator of first-degree burns from deeper ones that have not had time to blister. The classic first-degree injury is the sunburn or superficial scald burn from spills. These burns have no morbidity other than pain, and are therefore not calculated into burn size. Treatment includes oral pain medications, cool water compresses for the first day, and then application of any bland emollient to remoisturize the skin, such as aloe vera, cocoa butter, Eucerin cream, vitamin D, vitamin E, Aveeno, Lubriderm, and even Udder Butter, Bag Balm, or lard. Thicker ointments and those that are not quickly absorbed into the skin generally maintain lubrication for longer periods. Antimicrobial ointments need not be used on these burns.

Second-degree burns are synonymous with partial-thickness burns (those that burn only part way through the dermis). Epithelial elements remain in the undestroyed dermal appendages and spontaneous healing occurs in 7 to 28 days. Second-degree burns are very painful and are usually blistered. The blister fluid is clear and the underlying skin is wet and pink. The most common causes are spill scalds and flash burns. Treatment of these burns is protection with a biologic dressing. Deep partial-thickness burns are those that take more than 3 weeks to heal and have the potential to scar worse than grafted third-degree burns. If the patient's condition permits, these deeper burns are best treated with excision and skin grafting. When depth is uncertain or the burn is of mixed depth, these injuries are treated as third-degree burns, because biologic dressings generally do not adhere to these deeper wounds and provide little to no microbial control when not adherent.

Third-degree or full-thickness burns are those that extend through the dermis, destroying all epidermal and dermal elements. They require skin grafting for wound closure. When debrided, these burns appear deep red or white in color and are relatively insensate, although presence or absence of pain is an unreliable indicator of depth. They may initially have blisters containing hemorrhagic fluid. The resultant dead tissue is called *eschar* and must be removed before skin grafting. The prototype of these burns is the flame burn. Treatment is with topical antimicrobials and surgery.

Fourth-degree burns (deep burn necrosis) are those that extend into deep soft tissue, muscle, or bone such that closure with simple skin grafts is usually not possible. Electrical burns and deep thermal burns of the hands, anterior lower legs, and feet predominate (body parts where vital structures are very close to the skin surface). These burns often require surgical flap closure (free or pedicled) or extremity amputation.

Burn Size

Accurate initial assessment of burn size is essential for optimal patient care. Burn size is expressed as total body surface area (TBSA) or body surface area (BSA), wherein approximately 1% of a patient's surface area is equal to that of the palmar surface of the patient's hand with the fingers closed. This measurement is most useful for small (<5% TBSA) or spotty burns. For larger areas, the rule of nines (**Fig. 1**) provides a simple and rapid estimation of burn size in the adult. When calculating burn size using any method, first-degree burns are not counted and only the proportion of area actually burned is calculated. Thus, for an upper extremity to be considered 9% TBSA, the entire extremity from the shoulder to the finger tips must be burned at least to the blistering level. If only the posterior half of the upper extremity is burned, then burn size is considered to be 4.5% TBSA.

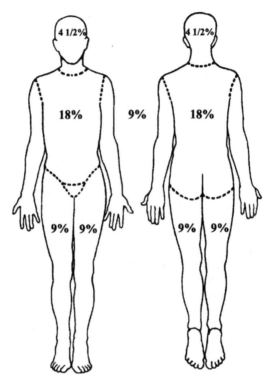

Fig. 1. Rule of Nines.

More accurate evaluation of burn size is made with a Berkow (**Fig. 2**) or Lund Browder chart, which identifies the different body proportions according to age of the patient (with children having larger heads and smaller lower extremities than adults) and through dividing the body into smaller units, such as dividing the upper extremity into the upper arm, lower arm, and hand (see **Fig. 2**). More recently, the use of computerized drawings simplifies calculations of size in both pediatric and adult patients and will even estimate fluid requirements. A version is also available for hand-held devices.[4]

Resuscitation

Fluid resuscitation is the cornerstone of early burn care. The microvascular structure beneath a burn wound develops increased permeability immediately after injury, which lasts through the first day post-burn. This capillary leak is up to molecular weight (MW) 30,000 d, effectively making the body two and a half fluid compartments instead of the normal three. The intravascular and extravascular extracellular compartments become one, except for the larger globulins and formed elements of the blood, which remain intravascular. This capillary leak is roughly directly proportional to burn size and becomes hemodynamically significant in burns larger than 20% TBSA (10% TBSA in young children or elderly patients). The objective of resuscitation is to replace this lost intravascular fluid with the minimal amount of fluid required to maintain normal bodily function.

Various formulas have been proposed to replace these fluids, which are either third spaced or completely lost into the burn dressing. These formulas replace

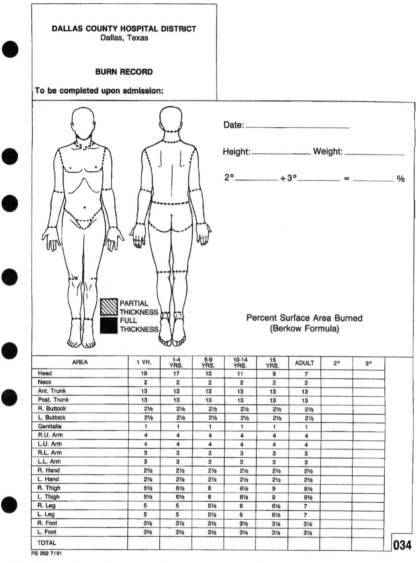

DALLAS COUNTY HOSPITAL DISTRICT
Dallas, Texas

BURN RECORD

To be completed upon admission:

Date: _____

Height: _____ Weight: _____

2° _____ +3° _____ = _____ %

PARTIAL THICKNESS

FULL THICKNESS

Percent Surface Area Burned
(Berkow Formula)

AREA	1 YR.	1-4 YRS.	5-9 YRS.	10-14 YRS.	15 YRS.	ADULT	2°	3°
Head	19	17	13	11	9	7		
Neck	2	2	2	2	2	2		
Ant. Trunk	13	13	13	13	13	13		
Post. Trunk	13	13	13	13	13	13		
R. Buttock	2½	2½	2½	2½	2½	2½		
L. Buttock	2½	2½	2½	2½	2½	2½		
Genitalia	1	1	1	1	1	1		
R.U. Arm	4	4	4	4	4	4		
L.U. Arm	4	4	4	4	4	4		
R.L. Arm	3	3	3	3	3	3		
L.L. Arm	3	3	3	3	3	3		
R. Hand	2½	2½	2½	2½	2½	2½		
L. Hand	2½	2½	2½	2½	2½	2½		
R. Thigh	5½	6½	8	8½	9	9½		
L. Thigh	5½	6½	8	8½	9	9½		
R. Leg	5	5	5½	6	6½	7		
L. Leg	5	5	5½	6	6½	7		
R. Foot	3½	3½	3½	3½	3½	3½		
L. Foot	3½	3½	3½	3½	3½	3½		
TOTAL								

PS 352 7/91

034

Fig. 2. Berkow chart. (*Courtesy of* Dallas County Hospital District, Dallas, TX; with permission.)

0.7 to 0.8 mEq of sodium per kilogram per percent burn in the first 24 hours, given at various rates and concentrations. The most commonly used formula is the Parkland formula, which suggests 4 mL of Ringer's lactate per kilogram of body weight per percent BSA burned during the first 24 hours post-burn. Using Ringer's lactate, electrolyte concentration is not a problem during resuscitation and values are not even measured. Underresuscitation is met with renal failure, hypotension, and multiple organ dysfunction, whereas overresuscitation results in pulmonary and cardiac overload and excessive edema formation. The extremes of age are especially sensitive to misestimation of fluid needs. Resuscitation requires an accurate estimation of the time of burn, burn size, and measurement of patient weight. Factors that increase fluid requirements include inhalation injury, late initiation of resuscitation, deep burns, acute intoxication, and preexisting malnutrition. All burn formulas are only starting points in resuscitation. Individual changes to fluid administration rates must be made hourly (or half-hourly in infants and small children) based on urine output and vital signs. Use of invasive vascular monitoring is seldom necessary. Non-burn fluid maintenance in children is added into the burn resuscitation as necessary, with maintenance in small children given as 5% dextrose/Ringer's lactate solution. Hypertonic resuscitation and timing for administration of colloids continue to be areas of research interest. All of the burn resuscitation formulas work well in experienced hands. The best formula is the one used by the burn center to which the patient is being transferred.

Inhalation Injury

Inhalation injury may be classified in several different ways, the simplest of which is division into carbon monoxide poisoning and upper and lower airway injuries.

Carbon monoxide is an odorless, tasteless gas that is very slightly lighter than air. It is produced by the incomplete combustion of carbon containing materials and causes more deaths in the United States than all other poisons.[5] It binds with hemoglobin in the red blood cell, forming carboxyhemoglobin (COHb), which has 210 times the bond for oxygen as normal hemoglobin, shifting the hemoglobin/oxygen dissociation curve to the left. In burn patients, the sometimes-subtle signs of cherry red lips or mucosa and symptoms of nausea and headache are absent, and therefore COHb levels should be measured in all patients who were trapped in a smoke-filled space. Optimal treatment is with 100% oxygen, which decreases the half-life of COHb from 4 hours to approximately 40 minutes. In the presence of elevated P_{AO_2} of COHb, measured and cutaneous saturations are meaningless. COHb levels do not correlate with patient outcomes.

Upper airway injury is a misnomer, and is really the result of swelling problems caused by external burns. These conditions do not necessarily imply pulmonary injury, because they also occur with scald burns. Edema formation in the posterior pharynx and glottic and subgottic areas associated with deep burns of the upper chest, neck, and lower face has the potential to catastrophically occlude the upper airway, most often at the level of the vocal cords in adults. Elevation of the head of the patient's bed helps minimize swelling until the airway is controlled. Upper airway stridor and increased work of breathing are very late signs of impending airway obstruction. Protection is accomplished through endotracheal intubation, with the tube carefully secured in place to avoid dislodgement once successfully placed. The endotracheal tube is left in position until swelling decreases to the point at which an airleak occurs when the tube cuff is deflated.

Lower airway or true smoke inhalation injury is caused by the patient inhaling the products of combustion, often as a result of being trapped in a closed space. Carbonaceous material is commonly suctioned from the airway. Fiberoptic bronchoscopy is the preferred diagnostic procedure. Early grading of inhalation injury severity is very inaccurate. The injury is basically a chemical burn from which resulting edema of the small airways creates distal microatelectasis and a clinical picture identical to acute respiratory distress syndrome (and with the same definition).[6] Significant injuries are those necessitating endotracheal intubation and mechanical ventilation for more than 4 days. Inhalation injury increases mortality for any given size burn and patient age.

BURN CENTER TRANSFER

Burn centers have been established that have a team of professionals dedicated to optimal burn care. The American Burn Association has established criteria for transfer of a patient to one of these centers (**Box 1**).[7]

Requirements for Transfer

Patients with major burns (>20% TBSA) require two large-bore peripheral intravenous lines that are securely sutured in position (burn exudate and rapidly changing extremity size from edema formation make conventional securing with tape or gauze wraps problematic). Catheters may be placed through the burned tissue. Central venous access should be avoided because of its high complication rate in the early post-burn period when vasospasm, low flow, and a hypercoagulable state contribute to complications. Intraosseous catheters may be placed as second choices in children. A urinary catheter and a nasogastric tube should be inserted. Use of ice on a burn wound is absolutely contraindicated because of the risk of a cold injury superposed on the burn. Continual efforts must be made to keep the patient warm. No burn debridement is required before transfer, and the burns should be wrapped in dry sterile or clean sheets and further covered with warm blankets. The general rule is that if the temperature is comfortable for the caregiver, it is cold for the burn patient.

Chemical Burns

A chemical burn is the only burn injury for which the care team can significantly impact severity. Appropriate use of personal protective equipment is mandatory. Beginning in the field, immediate irrigation with large volumes (gallons) of tap water is the preferred treatment for nearly all chemicals. The patient is completely unclothed and the bedding used during transport is changed. This procedure is followed by prolonged irrigation with tap water at a patient-selected temperature, with soap and a washcloth used to remove and dilute the remaining chemical. Neutralizing chemicals, such as sodium bicarbonate or acetic acid, should not be used to treat acid or alkali burns, respectively. Rarely, chemicals require special treatments, about which the local burn center should be contacted immediately. These include burns caused by hydrofluoric acid, phenol, and phosphorus. Burns caused by tar are scald burns, best cared for through dissolving the tar with a thick layer of neomycin ointment and then using an appropriate topical antimicrobial.

Electrical Burns

Electrical burns are the most devastating of burn injuries. These burns are more than skin-deep and often lead to amputations and long-term disabilities. A significant

---

Box 1
Criteria for burn center transfer

Partial-thickness burn greater than 10% TBSA

Third-degree burns in any age group

Burns involving the face, hands, feet, genitalia, buttocks, or major joints

Inhalation or traumatic injury

Electrical burns, including lightning injury

Chemical burns

number of these injuries become involved in the legal system, making accurate documentation essential. Electrocution is death by electricity. Thus, the injury in a living patient is better described as electrical shock or electrical burn. Likewise, the terms *entrance wounds* and *exit wounds* should be replaced by contact points, because most electrical burns are caused by a standard commercial 60 Hz alternating current that reverses direction 120 times per second.

Electrical burns are arbitrarily divided into low voltage (<1000 V), with minimal deep tissue injury, and high voltage (>1000 V), in which deep tissue (or hidden) injury is common. Arc burns are flash/flame burns caused by conversion of electricity into heat. These burns with or without current travel are treated as any other burn. Electrical burns have contact points that may have none, one, two, or many visible lesions. The scalp should be diligently searched for contact points hidden under the hair. Cardiac status is initially evaluated in the emergency department using a 12-lead EKG and continuous cardiac monitoring. In the presence of a normal EKG, prolonged (beyond the emergency room) cardiac monitoring is not necessary.[8]

Traumatic injuries occur at double the frequency with nonelectrical burns and must be evaluated appropriately. Red to brown to almost black pigmentation in the urine in the absence of hematuria is treated with mannitol (25 g) by intravenous push, followed immediately by two ampules of sodium bicarbonate, also by intravenous push, followed by Ringer's lactate at whatever rate is required to grossly clear the urine of pigment. Neurologic deficits occur frequently, and may occur or resolve within 2 years after the burn injury, thus mandating a complete neurologic examination on presentation.[9]

COMPARTMENT SYNDROMES

Formation of edema beneath full-thickness (usually circumferential) burn eschar has the potential to occlude arterial inflow to the extremity or restrict chest motion and hence ventilation. Treatment is with escharotomies performed at the bedside with either local anesthesia or conscious sedation. Incisions are placed mid-axially on the medial and lateral portions of affected extremities and on the mid-axillary lines of the trunk connected by an inverted "V" (chevron) incision along the costal margins.[10] Escharotomies of the fingers are seldom, if ever, required.

Muscle compartment syndromes are generally the result of electrical burns or extremely deep burns. Pain on passive stretch is the most consistent early sign, with loss of pulses occurring very late, after muscle death. Swollen, tight extremities in these situations mandate immediate and frequent serial clinical evaluations. Treatment is with multiple compartment fasciotomies of the affected extremities, performed in the operating room under general anesthesia.

WOUND CARE AND TOPICAL ANTIMICROBIALS

The nonviable burn wound (eschar) is a perfect medium for growth of bacteria, fungi, or viruses. The purpose of wound care is to debride necrotic tissue and remove previously applied topical agents, and to reapply new topical antimicrobials. Microbial flora are continually changing. The modern burn center is no longer the pseudomonas capital of the hospital. Dominant organisms depend on the specific burn center, but are presently often methicillin-resistant staphylococcous aureus and acinetobacter. Multiply resistant organisms complicate antibiotic choices. Prophylactic antibiotics are not indicated in burn patients. Burn wound cellulitis is usually treated with a first-generation cephalosporin antibiotic. Infected burns of the lower extremity in diabetic patients are first treated with a fluoroquinolone antibiotic.

Silver sulfadiazine is the most commonly used topical and is well tolerated with no side effects. It could be called "jack of all trades, master of none," having an intermediate spectrum and penetration. It has a very low allergic rate, and seldom is sulfa allergy a cause of avoidance. Enterobacter resistance is occasionally encountered. Silver sulfadiazine does not stain skin, nor does it cause leukopenia when used appropriately.[11] The authors use approximately 6.5 tons of silver sulfadiazine a year without need to change therapy.

Mafenide acetate (Sulfamylon) is a thick white cream that has an excellent effect against gram-negative organisms. It penetrates burn eschar to the extent that it is systemically absorbed, with it and its breakdown products being carbonic anhydrase inhibitors, which cause metabolic acidosis. Application is painful and approximately 10% of patients develop allergic reactions. It is best used for extremely deep burns, those infected with gram-negative organisms (especially pseudomonas), and for ear burns, in which its use along with a careful wound care program prevent chondritis, which can permanently destroy normal ear shape.[12] Sulfamylon solution (5%) is a clear liquid composed of mafenide acetate powder dissolved in normal saline. Its water-like characteristics make it an excellent topical agent to protect grafts and open wounds (without eschar). It does not cause metabolic acidosis, nor is pain or allergic reaction a problem.

Neomycin ointment is a bland topical agent that has only fair penetration and antibacterial coverage with minimal side effects. Uses include topical therapy for superficial burn wounds, fresh grafts, and also for the removal of solidified tar.

Silver nitrate is a 0.5% solution in water that, although it has an excellent antibacterial spectrum, does not penetrate eschar, causes hyponatremia and hypochloremic metabolic alkalosis, and stains everything it contacts gray or black. Its primary use is for graft protection on infected wound beds.

Recently, elemental silver has emerged as a convenient, effective, cost-saving topical agent. There has been significant focus on the sheet-type application of silver to partial-thickness burns, with products such as Aquacel Ag, Mepilex, and Silverlon offering convenience of easy application with the need for many fewer dressing changes and subsequent improved pain control. Clinical judgment is needed to appropriately determine the depth of the burn.

The combination of factors constituting current burn care has made burn wound sepsis a rare cause of death. Rather, death is now most often caused by pulmonary failure leading to multisystem organ failure.

Grafting

Skin grafting is the primary method of wound closure for third-degree burns. Before the 1970s, burn wounds were treated conservatively, with tanking of the patient. This procedure entailed immersion of the burned body parts and aggressive debridement with scissors, debriders, and even scalpels on a daily basis. After the underlying bed granulated, the wound was debrided in the operating room and skin grafted. In 1970, the Yugoslavian surgeon Zora Janzekovic[13] described what was then the revolutionary concept that full-thickness burn eschar did not have to undergo this 2- to 3-week process before grafting. Rather, she proposed early tangential excision of eschar with a knife with immediate application of skin graft onto the underlying viable fat bed. This technique is now standard of care in burn centers, with some early variation among burn centers, but usually beginning within 2 to 5 days post-burn. Tangential excision leaves normal tissue contours, but is associated with relatively high blood losses. Excision distal to pneumatic tourniquets prevents significant blood loss in extremity burns. In contrast, fascial excision of the burn wound carries the plane of tissue removal down to the relatively avascular subcutaneous tissue/fascia interface, where nearly bloodless surgery can be performed with electrocautery, but with significant cosmetic deformity and functional loss.

Skin grafts are harvested with a dermatome with thicknesses ranging from 0.006–0.014 inches (by comparison, a sheet of newspaper is approximately 0.003 inches thick). Graft thickness is selected based on burn size, patient age, and desired outcome. In general, what is good for the graft is bad for the donor site, and visa versa. Thus, thin split-thickness grafts have donor sites that heal rapidly and leave minimal scarring, although have poor cosmetic and functional graft results with significant graft contraction. Thick grafts undergo less contraction and have better appearance, but require donor sites that require longer time to heal and may scar worse than the graft. Meshing of skin grafts permits better conformance, take (through allowing blood, plasma, and bacteria to pass through the graft), and expansion, requiring less donor site area, although it is accomplished at the expense of worse cosmesis and more contraction, with associated longer graft healing times.

Donor site selection is planned to avoid crossing joints. Except for very large burns, the upper extremity below the elbow and lower extremity below the knee are generally avoided for cosmesis (and ease of ambulation in the latter case). The back provides a large area for graft harvesting but requires that the patient be turned under anesthesia. The scalp provides skin that is color-matched to the face and neck and provides a donor site normally hidden by hair, although at the expense of difficult harvesting from the complex convexity of the underlying skull.

Grafts are immobilized for 2 to 5 days, depending on graft location, patient cooperation, and cleanliness of the burn, with older, infected burns being undressed earlier and dependent areas with high shear forces, such as the back and buttocks, being taken down later.

Biologic Dressings and Skin Substitutes

Biologic dressings have extended wound care for individuals with both small and large burns. Pruitt and Levine[14] succinctly describe the necessary properties of skin substitutes. Although none of the available materials are perfect, their use is usually necessary for the care of patients with large burns (>50%–60% TBSA).

Allograft (also termed *homograft*, depending on whether Greek or Latin derivations are being used) is tissue obtained from another being of the same species. In the case of skin, it is obtained from human cadavers. Allograft continues to be the gold standard against which other biologic dressings are compared. Although usually available frozen (−160°F), the fresh form is used on large burns for better and longer adherence. Availability, quality, and cost are the primary limiting factors to its use. It may be placed over newly excised wounds or on top of widely expanded grafts for complete wound coverage. In the latter case, the allograft is allowed to separate spontaneously.

A xenograft (heterograft) is tissue obtained from a different species, which for skin is the pig. Porcine xenograft is available in several physical forms, such as meshed, unmeshed, rolls, and sheets, including 1 sq ft meshed sheets, which the authors prefer for convenience. This material provides 1- to 2-week coverage of partial-thickness burns, or temporary (days) coverage of excised burn wounds for which graft take is of concern. Heterograft adherence virtually assures excellent skin graft take on removal.

Synthetic dressings such as Biobrane, a nylon/silicone composite coated with porcine collagen, provide sterile, uniform sheets with minimal storage requirements.

Elastic properties of the material allow early movement of joints and changes in body part edema.

Biosynthetic dermal analogs (Integra) provide the cosmetic and functional advantages of thick grafts with thin donor sites. Disadvantages are expense and the need for two operations, the first for placement and the second for grafting with very thin split-thickness autografts approximately 2 weeks later (after vascularization of the neodermis). Cultured epithelial grafts in which a very small skin biopsy is expanded into a square meter or more of wound coverage may be necessary for care of very large burns. Limitations include very high expense, fragility, and high contraction rates. The ideal composite of cultured epidermis and dermis that could be placed in a single operation is not yet available.

Nutrition

Burns are the most hypermetabolic of all human injuries, with awareness of appropriate nutrition one of the important advances in modern burn care. No longer is the burn patient pictured as the malnourished victim of a prison camp. Provision of appropriate nutrition begins as soon as the patient arrives at the burn center, with placement of a feeding tube and continuous administration of enteral nutrition. Intragastric or postpyloric placement of the tube are both appropriate. Critically ill patients with controlled airways have their feeding continued up to and throughout surgery.

Daily requirements are calculated using the Harris-Benedict equation, with additions made for high stress, or measured using indirect calorimetry. The authors use relatively simple calculations, in which needs for burns over less than 20% TBSA are 30 to 35 kcal/kg with 1.5 to 2 g/kg protein and for larger burns (>20%) are 35 to 40 kcal/kg with 2 to 2.5 g/kg protein. All patients with major burn should be evaluated by a clinical dietician. Feeding usually involves standard commercially available formulations of 1 to 2 kcal/mL, with protein supplements as necessary. No evidence shows that additional special nutrition is beneficial. Stress ulceration is prevented with an H_2-blocker (ranitidine). Oxandrolone, an anabolic steroid analog, has been shown in a large multicenter trial to be of survival benefit for patients with large burns.[15] A portion of the burn hypermetabolism is often abrogated with the use of beta blockade. Although initially used for pediatric burns, its use has spread to the adult population.[16]

SUMMARY

Burn care begins with the moment of injury and continues until healing and scar maturation are complete.

REFERENCES

1. American College of Surgeons Committee on Trauma. Committee on trauma: advanced trauma life support. Chicago (IL): American College of Surgeons; 2008.
2. Advanced burn life support course. Available at: http://ameriburn.org/. Accessed January 8, 2011.
3. Lenoski E, Hunter K. Specific patterns of inflicted burn injuries. J Trauma 1977;17: 842–6.
4. SAGE II Surface Area Graphic Evaluation. SageDiagram, LLC, Free Ware. Available at: http://SageDiagram.com. Accessed January 8, 2011.
5. King M, Bailey C. Carbon monoxide–related deaths—United States, 1999–2004. MMWR Morb Mortal Wkly Rep 2007;56:1309–12.

6. Bernard G, Artigas A, Brigham K, et al. The American-European Consensus Conference on ARDS. Definitions, mechanisms, relevant outcomes, and clinical trial coordination. Am J Respir Crit Care Med 1994;149:818–24.

7. American Burn Association Burn Center Referral Criteria. Committee on trauma: resources for optimal care of the injured patient. Chicago (IL): American Burn Association, American College of Surgeons; 2006. p. 79–86. Available at: http://www.ameriburn.org. Accessed January 8, 2011.

8. Purdue G, Hunt J. Electrocardiographic monitoring after electrical injury: necessity or luxury. J Trauma 1986;26:166–7.

9. Petty P, Parkin G. Electrical injury to the central nervous system. Neurosurgery 1986;19:282–4.

10. Pruitt B, Dowling J, Montcrief J. Escharotomy in early burn care. Arch Surg 1968; 96:502–7.

11. Stiegler K, Hunt J, McDearmont S, et al. Reassessment of leukopenia associated with silver sulfadiazine use. J Burn Care Rehabil 2002;23(Suppl):S46.

12. Purdue G, Hunt J. Chondritis of the burned ear: a preventable complication. Am J Surg 1986;152:257–9.

13. Janzekovic Z. A new concept in the early excision and grafting of burns. J Trauma 1970;10:1103–8.

14. Pruitt B, Levine N. Characteristics and uses of biologic dressings and skin substitutes. Arch Surg 1984;119:312–22.

15. Wolf S, Edelman L, Kemalyan N, et al. Effects of oxandrolone on outcome measures in the severely burned: a multicenter prospective randomized double-blind trial. J Burn Care Rehabil 2006;27:131–9.

16. Herndon D, Hart D, Wolf S, et al. Reversal of catabolism by beta-blockade after severe burns. N Engl J Med 2001;345:1223–9.

Burn Wound Care

Karen J. Kowalske, MD

KEYWORDS
• Burn wound • Wound assessment • Dressings

The goals of burn wound care are removal of nonviable tissue, prevention of infection, and facilitation of wound healing, while controlling pain and maximizing outcome. This article reviews the basic pathophysiology of burn wounds; describes the evaluation of the depth, location, and extent of the wound; and discusses the myriad of wound care products on the market including their strengths and weaknesses. A burn clinician must remember that they are treating patients and not wounds and that adapting to the patient's individual circumstances is essential, including the type of wound and access to resources (ie, someone to change the dressing, a wound care product they can find and afford, and so forth). This article guides the reader through wound assessment and designing the appropriate treatment plan.

INITIAL ASSESSMENT

Burns cannot be managed without a direct visualization of the wound bed. Patients must be undressed and dressings must be removed. Even with direct visualization, it is quite difficult to determine wound depth initially. Many an expert clinician has been fooled on the initial evaluation.[1] Multiple technologies have attempted to circumvent this challenge including indocyanine green fluorescence, histologic assessment, and Doppler technology. Unfortunately, these are not cost effective and have no more accuracy than the expert clinician.[2] One of the ways around this is to have a good understanding of the mechanism of burn injury and the duration of hot contact, which can help determine the depth. In general, the hotter the substance and the greater the duration of contact, the deeper the burn. With a water temperature of 120°F, it takes in the range of 30 seconds to 10 minutes to obtain a full-thickness burn. With a temperature of 140°F to 150°F, it only takes a few seconds.[3,4] Water splash burns are not as deep as cheese sauce, which is not as deep as tar. Things that stick and dissipate heat into the skin create a deeper wound. Burns in patients with absent or decreased sensation tend to be full-thickness despite how they may appear initially.[5] The clinician must also be concerned if the pattern, depth, and mechanism of injury do not match. This is especially true for children, those with cognitive impairment, and the elderly.

This work was supported by funds from the National Institute on Disability and Rehabilitation Research, Office of Special Education and Rehabilitative Services, US Department of Education.
Department of Physical Medicine and Rehabilitation, University of Texas SW Medical Center, 5323 Harry Hines Boulevard, Dallas, TX 75390–9055, USA
E-mail address: karen.kowalske@utsouthwestern.edu

A story of a spill burn in a child with a water line mark consistent with being held under hot water requires referral to the appropriate authorities for investigation.

Wound assessment is based on color, degree of epithelial separation, and the coagulation of the eschar. Superficial (first degree) burns affect only the epidermis. This is essentially the depth of most sunburn. Individuals present with moderate pain and erythema without blistering. The redness resolves over a few days without any epithelial loss. Partial-thickness burns (second degree) involve the epidermis and part of the dermis. Superficial partial thickness is sunburn that peels. It heals without scarring within a week.[2] Mid partial-thickness burns effect about half of the dermal layer. This is a burn that blisters initially. There are numerous extensive reviews of whether these blisters should be unroofed or not (**Fig. 1**).[6] Leaving a blister intact decreases pain but may increase infection risk. In young children, it may make sense to leave the blister intact for the first few days to avoid discomfort. If the blister is opened by the clinician or if it opens spontaneously, an attempt can be made to get the separated epithelium to stick to the wound bed and act like a biologic dressing. As the wound epithelizes, the necrotic epithelium lifts off. This is an ideal way to limit pain and facilitate healing. This depth of burn takes about 2 weeks to heal and usually does not produce scarring but may result in pigmentation changes.

Deep partial-thickness burns involve the entire epidermis and dermis but spare the base of the hair follicle, which is lined with epithelial cells. It presents initially with nonadherent eschar. Once it is fully clean, numerous skin buds are visible (**Fig. 2**). This depth of burn is the most painful wound seen because of the exposed nerve endings associated with the skin buds. Although it heals spontaneously over about 3 weeks, the chaotic organization of the dermal matrix may lead to significant hypertrophic scarring.[2]

Full-thickness (third degree) burns present with a leathery appearance with well demarcated wound edges (**Fig. 3**). Hair, when pulled, slides out; thrombosed capillaries may be seen; and it has an adherent appearance. In general, a burn of this depth that is larger than the size of a quarter or in an area of important cosmesis or function,

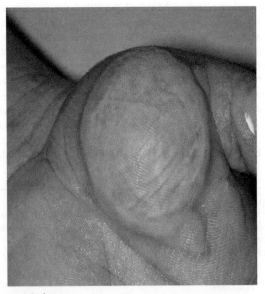

Fig. 1. Palmer blister at 3 days.

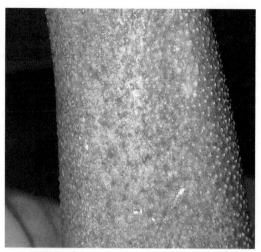

Fig. 2. Skin buds of a deep partial-thickness burn with exposed nerve endings are best soothed with silver sulfadiazine.

such as the back of the hand, requires skin grafting. These burns are mostly insensate because the nerve endings in the dermal layer have been lost but the clinician must remember that most burns are not a uniform depth and may have some areas of sparing of the nerve endings that can cause exquisite pain. Deep full-thickness (fourth degree) burns involve tendon, muscle, or bone. These wounds present with a charred or mummified appearance and amputation is universally required.[2]

PATHOPHYSIOLOGY

The burn wound can be divided into several zones. The central part of the wound, which had the most contact with the heat source, is the zone of coagulation in which cells are irreversibly damaged with no potential for regeneration. Immediately adjacent is the zone of stasis in which the cells have decreased blood flow but may be salvageable with fluid resuscitation and delicate wound care. Further ischemia or infection results in irreversible loss of this layer. The final zone is the zone of hyperemia. In

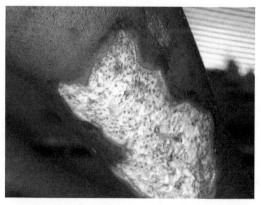

Fig. 3. Full-thickness wound with sharply demarcated edges and leathery adherent eschar.

this area, the cells have been inflamed but are not necrotic. The skin of these areas may look pink, which makes it difficult to determine if a patient has cellulitis. Marking these areas to look for progression over time may help with this determination. In response to the burn injury, the disrupted blood vessels in the outer two zones have increased capillary permeability, which results in water, protein, and electrolyte leak and edema formation. With circumferential injury on the chest or limbs, this pressure can create a tourniquet effect with resultant ischemia so close monitoring of tissue pressures may be warranted. This fluid loss continues until the skin surface has ree-pithelized. The fluid loss with resultant hemoconcentration can lead to capillary stasis and further ischemia of the wound bed.[5]

INITIAL WOUND CARE

Once the initial assessment has been completed, the wound needs to be cleaned thoroughly. Twenty years ago this wound care was done in a hydrotherapy tank. This language is still used today in the terms "hydro," "tanking," and "bathing" even though lowering patients into a tub of water is almost never done. Although many patients preferred the warmth of soaking, it was clear over time that the risks outweighed any potential benefits. Putting patients in water can result in hypothermia even if the water is relatively warm. Wound cross-contamination from one site to another can occur. Because, the fluid leak continues, it may worsen underlying hyponatremia.[7] Lastly, and probably the final straw, was that reimbursement for "tanking" is the same as for local care and the cost of filling, emptying, and cleaning the tanks made it fiscally impossible to continue this practice.

Modern wound care should be done in a designated area where strict infection prevention and control practices are mandated. The wound is washed with soap and water. Antibacterial soap and sterile water are not required. Using sterile technique the wounds are rinsed and scrubbed. The technique for rinsing can be gentle pouring of water over the wound or using a spray hose. Pulse lavage is painful and may over-debride, so is no longer commonly used. All topical agents and necrotic tissue should be removed. Often times, a straight edged razor, scissors, or forceps are required. In a facility, as much nonviable tissue as possible should be removed in each session. For patients doing their wound care at home a slower approach may be the pragmatic answer, removing only tissue that has clearly separated, because it takes an experienced professional to clearly differentiate viable from nonviable tissue, particularly in a wound of mixed depth.

TOPICAL AGENTS

Once the wound bed is clean the debate over the best topical agent or dressing begins. Unfortunately, there are actually relatively few good studies of the topical treatments of burn wounds.[8] Silver sulfadiazine (Silvadene; King Pharmaceuticals, Bristol, TN, USA) has been the mainstay of burn care for more than 40 years. Although there are many other wound care products on the market, a recent survey shows that most burn care experts continue to use silver sulfadiazine.[9] Wound healing may be a day or two slower with silver sulfadiazine compared with other agents.[10] Although sulfur allergy is a relative contraindication for silver sulfadiazine, most patients with a reaction to oral sulfonamides tolerate it without difficulty.[2] An occasional patient has a stinging sensation with silver sulfadiazine and those individuals should be switched to an alternative dressing. Glucose-6-phosphate dehydrogenase deficiency is a contraindication, because hemolysis can occur in these individuals.[5] Silver sulfadiazine can be applied with a tongue blade to the thickness of butter on bread (**Fig. 4**).

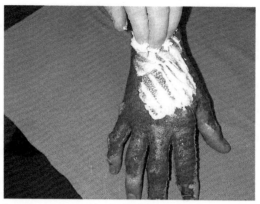

Fig. 4. Silver sulfadiazine is the mainstay of burn treatment and can be used for most wounds.

Dressings with silver sulfadiazine can stick to the wound bed, but this can be prevented by lightly impregnating the gauze with silver sulfadiazine at the time of application. If the dressing does stick, thoroughly wetting the dressing facilitates removal. Patients complain of slightly more pain than with other agents.[10] Although there was a theoretical concern about neutropenia, a large scale study showed no decrease in white blood counts in patients who received prolonged treatment with silver sulfadiazine.[11] Compared with other agents, the depth of penetration is less than ideal. It is bacteriostatic and it may impair epithelialization. So why do burn care providers continue to use silver sulfadiazine? It is widely available even in rural pharmacies; it is easy to apply; and it is generally soothing, particularly to exposed skin buds. Perhaps the main issue, however, is cost. At my own institution we use 2 tons of silver sulfadiazine per year to treat over 600 inpatients and more than a 1000 outpatients. That is 4000 lbs = 8800 kg. Our wholesale cost for silver sulfadiazine is $11 for a 400 g jar. That means we spend $2.42 million on silver sulfadiazine per year. If we switch to a wound care product that is $11 for 40 g then our costs go up $18 million dollars. Therefore, like other centers, we continue to use silver sulfadiazine for most wounds.

The second most common wound care agent selected by burn experts is antibiotic-impregnated gauze.[9] Although these products have also been shown to slightly slow time to full healing compared with other agents, they are readily available and easy to use. Triple antibiotic is available in almost any general store and is inexpensive and easy to use. These dressings have an even greater tendency to stick to the wound bed, which may damage newly healed epithelial cells. For large burns, single-ingredient antibiotic ointments are preferred to avoid the increase risk of allergic reaction associated with the use of a triple antibiotic ointment. For most burn units this agent is bacitracin. Mupirocin is usually reserved for treating patients with methicillin-resistant *Staphylococcus aureus* (MRSA).[2,5,12]

Mafenide acetate (Sulfamylon; Bertek Pharmaceuticals, Morgantown, WV, USA) has been commonly used in burns for many years. It has an excellent depth of penetration and provides broad-spectrum antimicrobial coverage but is not readily available outside of the burn unit and may produce a stinging sensation when used. The 5% solution is used on infected wounds or for very deep wounds.[13] Mafenide acetate cream is the agent of choice for full-thickness burns of the ears. It is somewhat expensive but the cost can be offset in areas that use large volumes.[2,13]

Acetic acid (0.25% solution) has been used in burn care. It is useful as a soak to decrease colonization with *Pseudomonas* but is usually not left on the wound because of excessive dryness.[2] Domboro solution (Bayer, Morristown, NJ, USA) can also be used in a similar way for controlling overgrowth of *Pseudomonas*.

BIOLOGIC DRESSINGS

Biologic dressings are temporary dressings that can decrease pain and fluid loss and facilitate wound closure. Xenograft (pigskin) is inexpensive and comes in large sheets. It is ideal for use over clean midpartial thickness wounds, such as chest scald burns in children (**Fig. 5**). It is left dry and eliminates the need for dressing changes. The healing epithelium pushes the xenograft off leaving healed skin underneath.[14,15] As it dries, it can give a pulling or tight sensation. If left on for more than 2 weeks, it can get incorporated into the skin and create a granulomatous phenomenon. If it is still adherent after 2 weeks, it can be coated with a thick layer of silver sulfadiazine, wrapped in gauze, and left overnight. The following day, the adherent xenograft separates off with soaking. Allograft (cadaveric skin) can be used on any partial-thickness burn but because of expense and the small size of the pieces, it is primarily reserved for chronic nonhealing wounds or to assess the viability of a full-thickness wound bed for accepting autograft.[16,17] Although it may remain in place for weeks, it is only a temporary coverage and must eventually be replaced with autograft. Autograft is the permanent coverage for large full-thickness wounds. Small wounds may close by epithelizing from the wound edges (see the article on acute care elsewhere in this issue).

SYNTHETIC DRESSINGS

A biosynthetic wound dressing sheet (Biobrane; Bertek Pharmaceuticals, Morgantown, WV, USA) has been used extensively and compares favorably with silver sulfadiazine in treating superficial partial-thickness burns. The downside for outpatient wound care is that it must be fully stretched and either stapled or steri-stripped into place. Therefore, it is usually applied in the operating room. It has been extensively used for donor site management (**Fig. 6**). The dressing can enclose dead tissue in the wound, providing a medium for bacterial overgrowth and invasive wound infection.[18–20]

A human fibroblast-derived temporary skin substitute (TransCyte; Smith & Nephew, Largo, FL, USA) has also been used on mid dermal burns after debridement and

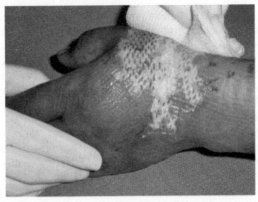

Fig. 5. Xenograft (pigskin) is moist when applied. It then dries out and separates from the underlying skin as it epithelizes.

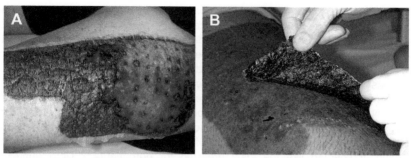

Fig. 6. (*A, B*) Biobrane on a donor site is wet initially. As it dries, it changes to a silvery color and can then be easily separated.

showed faster healing with less pain in two prospective trials.[21,22] The down side is that it is expensive and must be applied in the operating room and therefore has fallen quickly out of favor.

NONBIOLOGIC SYNTHETIC DRESSINGS

Compared with topical antibiotics, wound coverage with a synthetic dressing can lead to fewer dressing changes and less pain and anxiety for patients. These dressings include a contact layer dressing (Mepitel; Mölnlycke Health Care, Newtown, PA, USA) and a hydrocolloid (Duoderm; ConvaTec, Skillman, NJ, USA), which have shown to facilitate closure of small mid and superficial partial wounds.[19,23–25] Hydocolloid dressings (Duoderm) do not work on highly exudating wounds because the adhesive tends to separate. It can be used on wounds with adherent eschar for autolytic debridement. An occlusive biofilm (Tegaderm [3M, St Paul, MN, USA or Opsite [Smith-Nephew, Hull, UK]) has been used on partial-thickness wounds or donor sites, but if the wound has a high volume of exudates, the dressing separates and leaks onto the patients clothing. Most patients report that this dressing is soothing but they are frustrated when the seal separates.[26]

Petrolatum gauze (Xeroform; Kendall Healthcare, Mansfield, MA, USA) can be used to cover large areas of superficial burns (**Fig. 7**).[15] If petrolatum gauze does not adhere, the wound is likely deeper than suspected and should be treated with topical

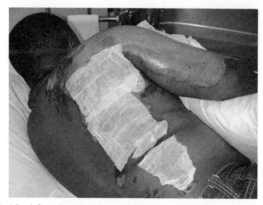

Fig. 7. Xeroform is ideal for clean mid partial-thickness burns or can be used in cut-to-fit patches for chronic wounds.

antibiotics or surgery. If it does adhere, it can be used like xenograft, kept dry and allowed to separate as the wound epithelizes. Fine mesh gauze is inexpensive but mostly only available at burn centers. This dressing can be allowed to adhere to the donor site with subsequent separation with epithelization or can be coated with anti-biotic ointment and used as a nonadherent dressing. Fine mesh can also be used on small areas of blistering to protect the fragile epithelium.

A nanocrystalline topical antibiotic gauze dressing coated with silver (Acticoat; Smith & Nephew, Largo, FL, USA) can be left on a wound for up to 7 days. This dressing may also be used over meshed skin grafts, and it seems to increase reepithelialization between the interstices of meshed grafts.[27] Because of the long wear time, it seemed like the ideal dressing for outpatients.[28] Unfortunately, it needs to be frequently moistened. If the dressing dries out it can be quite painful. The next dressing in this line is AquaCel (Conva Tec; Deeside, Flintshire, UK) Ag. It is a hydrofiber with impregnated silver. The advantage of this dressing is that it does not require frequent moisturizing and can be left in place for up to 14 days. The disadvantage is that it can be very adherent and is not easily removed for wound evaluation. Because of the adherence, some patients complain of pulling with movement.[29] The most recent evolution is a silver-impregnated adherent foam dressing (Mepilex Ag [Molnlycke, Norcross, GA, USA] or Contreet Foam [Coloplast, Humlebaek, Denmark]) (**Fig. 8**). This dressing is being used more frequently at burn centers for both partial- and full-thickness wounds. It is absorbent and tends to stay in place. It also controls bacterial overgrowth. Patients find this dressing quite soothing and it can be left in place for several days, which limits the labor needed for dressing changes. It is also easily removed for wound evaluation. The only down side of this product is its cost.[30]

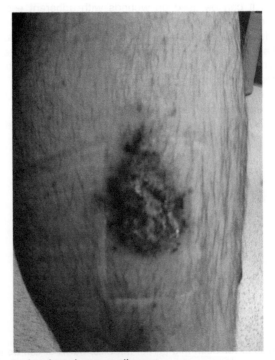

Fig. 8. Mepilex Ag is absorbent but nonadherent.

ENZYMATIC DEBRIDEMENT

Early debridement of burn eschar is beneficial to wound healing. Topical debridement products include collagenase and papain and can promote faster healing than silver sulfadiazine ointment.[15] Despite the theoretical advantage, enzymatic debridement results have been highly variable for both chronic wounds and burn wounds. The most recent addition to this market is the medical use of honey. This has shown promising results in both wound healing and to facilitate graft adherence.[31]

Nanofibers have been promoted as the next great evolution in wound care. A nanofiber matrix can mimic collagen fibers in the extracellular space to create a scaffold for wound healing and topical agents, culture cells, or other products can be added to facilitate wound closure. Unfortunately, early studies with these products have not shown promising results.[32]

FULL-THICKNESS BURNS

The goal in the management of full-thickness burns is the removal of the eschar and preparation of the bed for grafting. Silver sulfadiazine remains the mainstay of treatment for full-thickness burns along with continuing debridement. Any of the other dressings outlined previously can also be used as a temporary covering before grafting. Allograft (cadaver skin) is only available in small pieces and is relatively expensive. Most reserve this product for bed preparation before grafting in chronic nonhealing wounds or in patients with large surface area burns to make sure the bed is ready for autografting.[2,5]

FRESH SKIN GRAFT

The traditional approach for autografts is to cover them with a thin layer of antibiotic ointment. Other options include Xeroform (Covidien, Mansfield, MA, USA) or nonadherent gauze. Recent studies support the use of topical assisted negative pressure to facilitate graft vascularization of relatively avascular wound beds (see the article on acute care elsewhere in this issue).[33]

DONOR SITES

Donor sites are a classic mid partial-thickness wound. Because, they are symmetric in shape and depth, this provides an excellent opportunity for comparing wound treatments. Silver sulphadiazine is still frequently used but requires daily dressing changes. Biobrane can be used because it can be stapled down in the operating room. As the bed heals, it converts to a silver, color which helps the clinician and patient know when to facilitate separation. Film (Tegederm) sealed dressings work well on small sites but when used on the thigh there is a tendency to separate. Patients then complain about the drainage onto clothing. Dressings that dry out and become adherent, such as xenograft, Xeroform, or fine mesh, are inexpensive and easy to use but initially are quite painful. Acticoat seemed like an ideal dressing initially but it needs to be kept adherent until the wound bed heals. Current trials are being done with foam dressings (Mepilex Ag), which seems like a promising alternative.

EXPOSED TENDONS

The most common exposed tendon is the extensor mechanism of the finger. The hand is a common location for burn injuries and the dorsal skin is very thin. Managing this exposed tendon is critically important for maximizing function of the hand. The extensor mechanism is fragile and can easily dry out, rupture, and produce a Bouti-nerre deformity. This tendon can be kept moist by using 2nd skin (Spenco, Waco, TX, USA), which is a hydrogel dressing that keeps the tendon moist (**Fig. 9**). If this is not available, a thick layer of antibiotic ointment can keep the tendon moist. Drying agents should never be used over an exposed tendon. Negative pressure therapy may also be considered to improve vascularization of the wound bed.[34] Overstretch of the tendon should be avoided (see the article on hand care elsewhere in this issue). The Achilles tendon is also commonly exposed. This can be immobilized using a total contact sandal with a molded upright. Because the tendon is so thick, it is less likely to tear fully but it still should be protected. Using a sterile needle and pin pricking around the edge can facilitate granulation. A few needle sticks through the tendon also can facilitate a blood supply through the tendon. Exposed tendons of the forearm can be protected by immobilizing the wrist in a standard splint. Overstretch should be avoided to prevent rupture.

EXPOSED BONE

With an isolated injury and exposed bone, a rotation flap or free flap is ideal. Unfortu-nately, exposed bone following burn injury is often associated with significant tissue loss locally prohibiting rotational flap and the surrounding scarring may prohibit free flap. Because the exposed bone is relatively avascular, osteomyelitis is rare. Exposed tibia can be treated with pin pricking around the edges just as is done with exposed tendons. Another option is surgical burr holes into the bone. Following this procedure, a sterile needle can be used to facilitate the migration of marrow cells, which differen-tiate into granulation cells and provide a vascular cellular base for epithelialization (**Fig. 10**). Exposed bone digit tips and larger areas of mummification are kept dry and the edges are treated with an appropriate topical. Eventually the exposed tip of mummified tissue needs to be resected.

CHRONIC WOUNDS

Nonhealing wounds are a significant challenge in wound care. Most wounds heal, so in assessing the nonhealing wound one must review the causes of slow healing including avascularity, infection, tissue trauma, and overall nutritional status. There is usually not

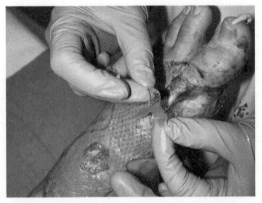

Fig. 9. 2nd skin is used on exposed tendons, which must be kept moist to avoid tendon rupture.

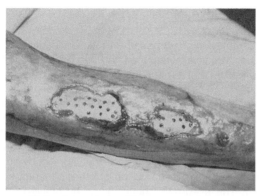

Fig. 10. Exposed bone with fresh burr holes. The marrow migrates out and creates a bed of granulation to facilitate epithelization.

significant eschar, so vigorous debridement is not required. Areas of hypergranulation should be treated with silver nitrate sticks. Areas of avascularity may require treatment with course gauze. The most common culprit of infection is MRSA or *Pseudomonas*. For MRSA, topical treatment with mupirocin is the initial approach. Other options include half-strength betadine, or Xeroform patches cut to fit the open wound bed can be allowed to stick to the wound and separate as the wound epithelizes (**Fig. 11**). If the patches come off, they should be replaced. If the patches repeatedly do not adhere, additional antibiotic treatment may be required. For *Pseudomonas*, acetic acid, Domboros, or manefide soaks can facilitate wound closure. Silver nitrate sticks are used in hypergranulated wound beds. Epithelial cells cannot grow uphill, so the edges of the wound should be cauterized with silver nitrate to facilitate closure.

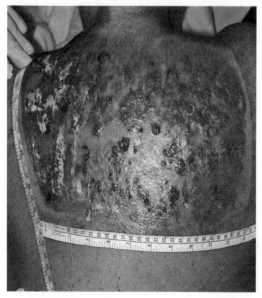

Fig. 11. Chronic wounds require gentle care to avoid traumatizing fragile epithelial regrowth.

ANATOMIC CONSIDERATIONS
Head

The general approach to the face and head is to use antibiotic ointment. Silver sulfa-diazine tends to liquefy when warm and then drip. Also, it is quite irritating to the eyes. Facial debridement should not be too vigorous to avoid traumatizing the fragile tissues. The hair follicles harbor bacteria making these areas prone to prolonged heal-ing and repeated breakdown (**Fig. 12**). Shaving the involved areas can keep the hair follicles from interfering with wound healing but can also traumatize the healing tissues. Gently washing once per day is recommended. Debridement should only be done when absolutely necessary to avoid traumatizing the tissues. Scabs should be removed only when they are purulent and draining. Antibiotic ointment is used on the eyebrows to facilitate separation of tar or other adherent substances without manual debridement. The eyebrows should never be shaved because of the risk that the hair may not regrow. Lips and eyelid burns are almost never full thickness. Because of the nature of the tissues, they should not be aggressively debrided but rather they should be gently washed. They also dry out easily, so it is important to keep them very moist. Antibiotic ointment can be used but tastes bad. The provider should consider using petroleum jelly. Camphor products should be avoided because they have a tendency to be irritating.

Ears

Silver sulfadiazine tends to liquefy when warm and can cause external otitis. Because the ear cartilage is relatively avascular, mafenide acetate (Sulfamylon) is a better choice. It has an increased depth of penetration and is more the consistency of

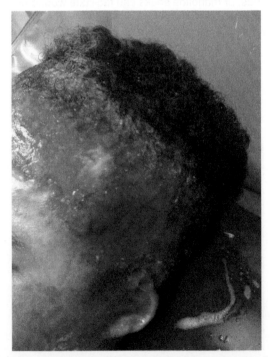

Fig. 12. Removing eschar on the scalp should be limited to avoid enlarging the wound and traumatizing the cells. Trimming the hair facilitates wound closure.

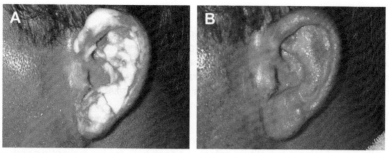

Fig. 13. (*A, B*) Mafenide acetate works well on the ears because of its depth of penetration and consistency.

toothpaste so it conforms and stays in place on the ear. For more superficial wounds, antibiotic ointment can be used. It must be noted that the ear can develop an inflammatory response to topical agents, called pseudochondritis. With this condition, there is increased swelling and drainage. Although it is tempting to switch the topical or start intravenous antibiotics, the first approach should be to remove all topicals for at least 24 hours to see if the ear improves (**Fig. 13**).

LUBRICATION

Once the burn wounds are epithelized, lubrication is essential to avoid repeated breakdown. Products without alcohol or perfume are preferred. Frequent reapplication is essential to avoid cracking and decrease the risk of shear injury (**Fig. 14**). It has also been shown that frequent moisturizing decreases the development of hypertrophic scarring. No specific product has been proved better than other products. Whatever lubricant the patient buys into and agrees to frequently apply is the best answer.

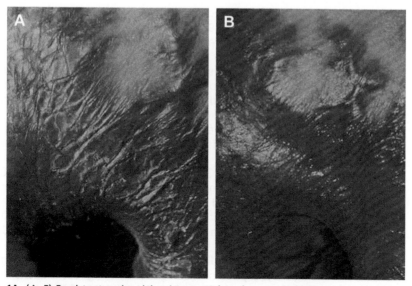

Fig. 14. (*A, B*) Persistent moisturizing is essential to decrease itching.

SUNSCREEN

Waterproof sunscreen is recommended until the tissue has returned to its preburn color. Any agent with a sun-protection factor greater than 15 should be adequate but must be reapplied at a minimum of every 2 hours when the patient is outdoors. Clothing provides a natural sun protection. Only rarely is sun-protective clothing required. Surprisingly, once the scar tissue is mature, it can tolerate some sun exposure.

SUMMARY

Wound care involves cleansing with soap and water, and application of a topical agent or a synthetic or biologic substitute selected specifically for the patient's needs. Each wound should be evaluated specifically for depth and location so that the care can be individualized with specific attention paid to the pragmatic aspects of costs and the need for dressing changes. Most partial-thickness burns heal with almost any intervention so the most expensive agents are not always required. Full-thickness burns usually need to be grafted. Lubrication and sun protection are essential once the wound is healed.

REFERENCES

1. Heimbach JT, Orwin RG. Public perceptions of sodium labeling. J Am Diet Assoc 1984;84:1217–9.
2. Johnson RM, Richard R. Partial-thickness burns: identification and management. Adv Skin Wound Care 2003;16:178–87 [quiz: 88–9].
3. Katcher ML. Tap water scald prevention: it's time for a worldwide effort. Inj Prev 1998;4:167–8.
4. Moritz AR, Henriques FC Jr. The reciprocal relationship of surface temperature and time in the production of hyperthermic cutaneous injury. Am J Pathol 1947;23:897.
5. Merz J, Schrand C, Mertens D, et al. Wound care of the pediatric burn patient. AACN Clin Issues 2003;14:429–41.
6. Richard R, Johnson RM. Managing superficial burn wounds. Adv Skin Wound Care 2002;15:246–7.
7. Said RA, Hussein MM. Severe hyponatraemia in burn patients secondary to hydrotherapy. Burns Incl Therm Inj 1987;13:327–9.
8. Wasiak J, Cleland H, Campbell F. Dressings for superficial and partial thickness burns. Cochrane Database Syst Rev 2008;4:CD002106.
9. Hermans MH. Results of an Internet survey on the treatment of partial thickness burns, full thickness burns, and donor sites. J Burn Care Res 2007;28:835–47.
10. Stern HS. Silver sulphadiazine and the healing of partial thickness burns: a prospective clinical trial. Br J Plast Surg 1989;42:581–5.
11. Thomson PD, Moore NP, Rice TL, et al. Leukopenia in acute thermal injury: evidence against topical silver sulfadiazine as the causative agent. J Burn Care Rehabil 1989;10:418–20.
12. Ovington LG. The truth about silver. Ostomy Wound Manage 2004;50:1S–10S.
13. Kucan JO, Smoot EC. Five percent mafenide acetate solution in the treatment of thermal injuries. J Burn Care Rehabil 1993;14:158–63.
14. Chatterjee DS. A controlled comparative study of the use of porcine xenograft in the treatment of partial thickness skin loss in an occupational health centre. Curr Med Res Opin 1978;5:726–33.
15. Hansbrough W, Dore C, Hansbrough JF. Management of skin-grafted burn wounds with Xeroform and layers of dry coarse-mesh gauze dressing results in excellent graft take and minimal nursing time. J Burn Care Rehabil 1995;16:531–4.

16. Eldad A, Din A, Weinberg A, et al. Cryopreserved cadaveric allografts for treatment of unexcised partial thickness flame burns: clinical experience with 12 patients. Burns 1997;23:608–14.

17. Vloemans AF, Middelkoop E, Kreis RW. A historical appraisal of the use of cryopreserved and glycerol-preserved allograft skin in the treatment of partial thickness burns. Burns 2002;28(Suppl 1):S16–20.

18. Barret JP, Dziewulski P, Ramzy PI, et al. Biobrane versus 1% silver sulfadiazine in second-degree pediatric burns. Plast Reconstr Surg 2000;105:62–5.

19. Cassidy C, St Peter SD, Lacey S, et al. Biobrane versus duoderm for the treatment of intermediate thickness burns in children: a prospective, randomized trial. Burns 2005;31:890–3.

20. Hansbrough JF. Use of Biobrane for extensive posterior donor site wounds. J Burn Care Rehabil 1995;16:335–6.

21. Demling RH, DeSanti L. Management of partial thickness facial burns (comparison of topical antibiotics and bio-engineered skin substitutes). Burns 1999;25:256–61.

22. Noordenbos J, Dore C, Hansbrough JF. Safety and efficacy of TransCyte for the treatment of partial-thickness burns. J Burn Care Rehabil 1999;20:275–81.

23. Gotschall CS, Morrison MI, Eichelberger MR. Prospective, randomized study of the efficacy of Mepitel on children with partial-thickness scalds. J Burn Care Rehabil 1998;19:279–83.

24. Hermans MH. HydroColloid dressing (Duoderm) for the treatment of superficial and deep partial thickness burns. Scand J Plast Reconstr Surg Hand Surg 1987;21:283–5.

25. Afilalo M, Dankoff J, Guttman A, et al. DuoDERM hydroactive dressing versus silver sulphadiazine/Bactigras in the emergency treatment of partial skin thickness burns. Burns 1992;18:313–6.

26. Poulsen TD, Freund KG, Arendrup K, et al. Polyurethane film (Opsite) vs. impregnated gauze (Jelonet) in the treatment of outpatient burns: a prospective, randomized study. Burns 1991;17:59–61.

27. Demling RH, Leslie DeSanti MD. The rate of re-epithelialization across meshed skin grafts is increased with exposure to silver. Burns 2002;28:264–6.

28. Varas RP, O'Keeffe T, Namias N, et al. A prospective, randomized trial of Acticoat versus silver sulfadiazine in the treatment of partial-thickness burns: which method is less painful? J Burn Care Rehabil 2005;26:344–7.

29. Caruso DM, Foster KN, Blome-Eberwein SA, et al. Randomized clinical study of Hydrofiber dressing with silver or silver sulfadiazine in the management of partial-thickness burns. J Burn Care Res 2006;27:298–309.

30. Karlsmark T, Agerslev RH, Bendz SH, et al. Clinical performance of a new silver dressing, Contreet Foam, for chronic exuding venous leg ulcers. J Wound Care 2003;12:351–4.

31. Jull AB, Rodgers A, Walker N. Honey as a topical treatment for wounds. Cochrane Database Syst Rev 2008;4:CD005083.

32. Hromadka M, Collins JB, Reed C, et al. Nanofiber applications for burn care. J Burn Care Res 2008;29:695–703.

33. Moiemen NS, Yarrow J, Kamel D, et al. Topical negative pressure therapy: does it accelerate neovascularisation within the dermal regeneration template, Integra? A prospective histological in vivo study. Burns 2010;36:764–8.

34. Heugel JR, Parks KS, Christie SS, et al. Treatment of the exposed Achilles tendon using negative pressure wound therapy: a case report. J Burn Care Rehabil 2002;23:167–71.

Positioning, Splinting, and Contracture Management

William S. Dewey, PT[a],*, Reg L. Richard, MS, PT[a],
Ingrid S. Parry, MS, PT[b]

KEYWORDS

• Splinting • Positioning • Contracture • Burn • Scar

The development of burn scar contracture is a pathologic condition. Burn scar contracture is defined as a loss of motion of a joint or anatomic structure as a result of normal skin being replaced by inextensible scar tissue.[1] The presence of a burn scar contracture has been shown to have a negative impact on a burn survivor's quality of life, particularly in regards to physical functioning.[2] A focus of burn rehabilitation should be to prevent or minimize contractures of the affected areas. Based on biomechanical considerations (discussed later), appropriate splinting and positioning is a critical component of any comprehensive burn rehabilitation program designed to attain optimal range-of-motion (ROM) outcomes. In 2008, a schema of burn rehabilitation phases (acute, intermediate, and long term) was developed to delineate the components of burn care treatment that are emphasized at different points in the continuum of care (**Fig. 1**).[3] **Table 1** describes the primary goals for positioning and splinting of burn patients during each burn rehabilitation phase.

BIOMECHANICS

Biologic tissue adapts to the mechanical influences of applied external forces. Placing stress on tissue can cause it to change shape or form.[4] Excessive stress causes

The authors have nothing to disclose.

The opinions or assertions contained herein are the private views of the author and are not to be construed as official or as reflecting the views of the Department of the Army, the Department of Defense, or Shriners Hospitals for Children.

[a] U.S. Army Burn Center Rehabilitation Department, U.S. Army Institute of Surgical Research, 3400 Rawley E. Chambers Avenue, Building 3611, Fort Sam Houston, San Antonio, TX 78234-6315, USA

[b] Shriners Hospital for Children—Northern California, 2425 Stockton Boulevard, Sacramento, CA 95817, USA

* Corresponding author.

E-mail address: scott.dewey@amedd.army.mil

Phys Med Rehabil Clin N Am 22 (2011) 229–247

doi:10.1016/j.pmr.2011.02.001

1047-9651/11/$ – see front matter. Published by Elsevier Inc.

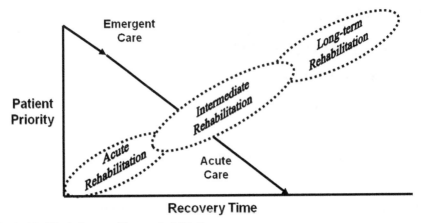

Fig. 1. Modified phases of burn rehabilitation.

damage to the tissue while too little stress is insufficient to stimulate change beyond normal cellular turnover. When treating patients with burn injury, splinting or positioning interventions must strike a stress balance to be effective. Developing an understanding of the biomechanic principles that underlie these physical interventions in the management of burn scar contracture aids in improving burn rehabilitation practice, leading to improved patient outcomes.

Both skin and scar tissue are comprised of an extracellular matrix—a solid fibrous network with a viscous liquid component, herein referred to as ground substance. In natural skin, collagen and elastic fibers provide integrity and elasticity, respectively. These components interact to protectively limit extensibility and provide tissue recoil after elongation. In contrast, burn scar tissue is only composed of collagen fibers within an altered ground substance environment and elastic fibers are absent. The collagen fibers are arranged in no predictable pattern. The predominant subcomponent of ground substance is chondroitin sulfate A, a substance found in abundance in bone tissue. This biologic composition of burn scar tissue is thought to be a possible cause of the inextensibility seen in burn scar.

With joint movement, skin or scar needs to accommodate to a change in limb length.[5,6] As limb length increases, collagen fibers unfurl and orient in the direction of force applied. As skin, more so than scar, is elongated further, additional collagen fibers sequentially align in the direction of the force applied. As collagen fibers move, the ground substance is displaced from between the fibrous network. When movement is reversed, the collagen fibers retract to their normal resting position while again having to redisplace the surrounding ground substance.

Successive length induction (SLI) or preconditioning of tissue, commonly referred to as stretching tissue, is an important concept to enlist whether fabricating a splint or setting up a positioning program for a patient. SLI entails repeatedly elongating a tissue

Table 1	
Positioning and splinting goals for each burn rehabilitation phase	
Phase of Rehabilitation	**Goal**
Acute	Edema control and pressure relief
Intermediate	Tissue elongation and graft protection
Long term	Tissue elongation

until it reaches its safe maximal length (**Fig. 2**). Maximal length of tissue has been reported to occur after 7 to 9 repetitions up to a tissue's yield point (**Fig. 3**).[7] In a clinical situation, however, the yield point of tissue is rarely reached due to pain complaints in conscious patients. Safe, maximal preconditioning of tissue can be clinically determined when a patient's ROM about a given joint ceases to increase with repeated repetitions. When preparing to fabricate or apply a splint, it is ideal to employ SLI until the tissue has achieved its maximal preconditioned length. At end range, this causes the tissue to be under tension. When tension is removed, tissue naturally retracts back to its desired resting length. Loading and unloading of tissue when plotted on a stress-strain curve produces a hysteresis type of pattern (see **Fig. 2**). With each successive lengthening, more and more ground substance is displaced from between the compacted fibers. The delay in tissue retraction is attributed to redistribution of the ground substance. It is important, however, to remember that all tissue wants to remain at its resting length. Much research is still needed in the area of biomechanics related to the burn injured population. Understanding basic biomechanical principles when applying rehabilitation techniques, however, helps burn therapists better understand the expected response to treatment.

Biomechanical principles can be applied when deciding on the appropriate positioning or splinting device to provide a lengthening force to a burn scar. If the device applies a static force, the biomechanical principle of stress relaxation is involved (**Fig. 4**). Before fabricating a splint, tissue surrounding the splinted joint of interest should be preconditioned to achieve an optimal length and the splint fabricated to maintain that length. The amount of tension felt by a patient decreases as the tissue accommodates to this extended length. Each time such force is applied (the static splint is donned), a patient's tissue may need to be preconditioned in order for the splint to fit properly again. Therefore, based on the principle of tissue stress relaxation, patients initially should be splinted or positioned with their tissue under tension knowing that the amount of tension will subside to a more comfortable level because the force over time required to maintain the tissue at a given length is reduced. Similarly, serial static and static progressive types of splints repeatedly harness stress relaxation of tissue or the principle of tissue creep (discussed later), depending on the interval of time between adjustments.

Tissue creep is another biomechanical principle used when splinting burn patients. Different from stress relaxation, tissue creep applies a constant force to progressively lengthen tissue over time (**Fig. 5**). This type of tissue reaction is seen with the use of dynamic splints. Dynamic splints commonly use elastic bands or springs to apply

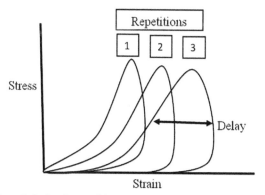

Fig. 2. Successive length induction and hysteresis.

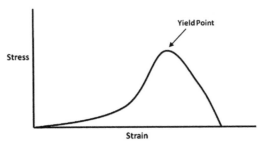

Fig. 3. Stress-strain curve.

constant tension to tissue. As tissue lengthens, the constant force causes the tissue to lengthen further by biologic adaptation through tissue growth. Tissue expanders used in burn reconstructive procedures are another example of the application of tissue creep.

POSITIONING

The position of comfort after burn injury is typically the position that promotes deformity and therefore should be avoided. Suggested anticontracture positioning can be found in the literature.[8–10] Common anticontracture positioning has been described as follows: neck in extension, shoulder abducted to 90 to 110° and horizontally adducted 15 to 20° or in the position of scaption,[9–11] elbow extension, forearm supination, wrist extension of 15 to 25° with neutral deviation, MCP joints in 60 to 70° flexion, interphalangeal (IP) joints in extension, thumb in palmar abduction, hip extension and abducted 20° (no external rotation), knee extension, and neutral ankle dorsiflexion.[8–10] There is no universal position, however, to prevent all contractures,[8] and burn depth and location must be considered when determining optimal anticontracture positioning. Positioning is also used for managing edema, facilitating functional alignment of joints, enabling wound care, and preventing peripheral neuropathies.[1] Positioning may be active, which is nonrestrictive and ideal for cooperative patients, or passive, which involves the use of restraints or splinting.[12] Positioning protocols must be monitored regularly for effectiveness and require cooperation of the entire burn team for successful implementation.

SPLINTING
Indications

Although splint use varies among burn rehabilitation professionals,[13–17] it is a common intervention used to prevent scar contractures.[1,14] Splints are used through all phases of burn rehabilitation[1,14–17] with indications being soft tissue or skin graft protection,

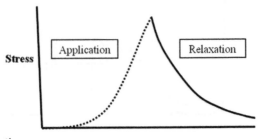

Fig. 4. Stress relaxation.

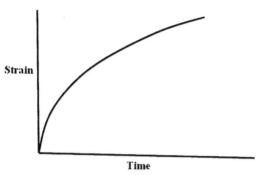

Fig. 5. Tissue creep.

antideformity positioning, tissue lengthening, or tissue length preservation.[1,18] Early implementation of splints is a key component of contracture management because of the influence on collagen orientation of developing fibers.[3,19,20] Burn scar contractures may be perceived as a late sequella of a burn; however, burn scar contractures begin with the process of wound closure and continue through scar maturation. Applying current statistical analysis, Huang and colleagues[21] and Bunchman II and colleagues[22] demonstrated a decreased contracture rate when using splints compared with not using splints (**Table 2**). Patients who wore splints for more than 6 months had less chance of developing a scar contracture than those who wore splints for a shorter period of time.[21,22] Additionally, a preliminary report showed that splinting interventions can reverse scar contractures more rapidly compared with routine interventions, including exercise, massage, and pressure in the long-term rehabilitation phase.[23]

Types

There are 3 types of splints routinely used with burn patients: static splints, static progressive splints, and dynamic splints.[1] Static splints maintain a fixed position and are indicated for skin graft protection after surgery or anticontracture positioning if adequate ROM is not gained with exercise alone. Static splints can be serially modified to account for increased tissue length gained with exercise or extended positioning.[8] Static progressive splints or dynamic splints are indicated if sufficient ROM is not obtained with static positioning and exercise. Such splints may be implemented for correction of contractures. Static progressive splints provide inelastic stress to tissue at end range and allow adjustment to the stress as the tissue lengthens via stress relaxation.[1,24] Dynamic splints provide a continual stress to tissue over

Table 2										
Odds ratio describing contracture versus no contracture										
Splint	**Axilla**		**Elbow**		**Wrist**		**Knee**		**Neck**[a]	
Time	**OR**	**P Value**	**OR**	**P Value**	**OR**	**P Value**	**OR**	**P Value**	**OR**	**P Value**
<6 mo	2.04	0.25	1.9	0.09	0.8	0.38	2.9	0.04	5.4	<0.01
6–12 mo	14.5	<0.01	8.8	<0.01	3.9	<0.01	9.8	<0.01		
>12 mo	38.6	<0.01	18.9	<0.01	6.6	<0.01	14.7	<0.01		

Abbreviation: OR, odds ratio.
[a] Specific time frame not stated.

time.[1,25] A hierarchical approach to splinting has been advocated that suggests the use of static progressive splinting for more restrictive tissue shortening and dynamic splinting for more responsive tissue deficits.[26] The use of well-designed static progressive or dynamic splints obviates remolding the basic form of the splint as is done with serial static splinting. Instead, the straps, slings, hinges, or other mobile forces can be modified as motion changes. A case study showed increased ROM when using a dynamic splint compared with a static splint.[25] Many splint designs have been described in the literature[27,28]; however, there are minimal studies comparing the effectiveness of these devices. Thus, prospective randomized comparative studies are needed to identify optimal splinting practices (**Fig. 6**).[1]

Dynamic and static progressive splints are both commercially available and can be custom fabricated. Advantages of custom-fabricated splints are that they can accommodate to a patient's unique size and profile and can be adjusted as edema fluctuates or bandage thickness changes. Disadvantages of custom-fabricated dynamic or static progressive splints are that they can be technically challenging and can be time consuming to fabricate. Some of the technical challenges pertain to the direction of pull on the involved body part(s). The angle of pull should be 90° to prevent friction and provide an optimal force.[29] Splint adjustments have to be made continuously to maintain this angle of pull as ROM gains are made. The force should remain a low-load force as previously indicated.

Principles

Regardless of the splint type, some basic principles should be considered when fabricating and applying splints: (1) splint design should be simple; (2) wound depth and available ROM should be considered; (3) splint should accommodate skin recruitment throughout cutaneous functional units[6]; (4) instruction on splint indications, precautions, wearing schedule, and proper fit should be given to the patients and care providers; (5) splint fit should be re-evaluated regularly; (6) hands should be given special consideration due to the complex anatomic implications; (7) adequate time should be allotted for splint fabrication; and (8) an optimal splint wearing schedule should be monitored and modified based in patient response.[14]

Splint design

A device is only effective if fabricated and applied properly. Although complexity may be necessary with multiple joint involvement, ensuring that patients and/or care providers are able to properly apply a splint so the device can be worn without compromising its primary purpose is an important education piece. Generally speaking, static splints should be attempted before more complex dynamic or static progressive splinting.

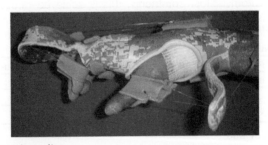

Fig. 6. Static progressive splint.

Wound depth and ROM considerations

Superficial partial-thickness burns typically do not require splinting due to the low contracture risk associated with rapid reepithelialization.[1] A splint is highly recommended for deep partial-thickness or full-thickness burns if patients are unable to achieve full active ROM, have impaired consciousness, or are noncompliant with their exercise program.[1] Splints should also be considered to immobilize joints where exposed tendons are present to protect these structures from rupture.

Splints and cutaneous functional units

Fields of skin recruited during ROM must be considered when contemplating which joints should be included in a splint.[6] Although skin closest to the involved joint is of particular interest, skin is still recruited serially as ROM increases.[6] If ROM of a particular joint is more limited when an adjacent joint is moved into a position requiring greater tissue length, then both joints should be included in the splint. This places the involved tissue in a lengthened position to provide optimal tissue stress.

Splint instruction for patients and care providers

Patients or care providers must have a good understanding of the purpose for a splint and a proper wearing schedule to facilitate compliance. Caregivers should be instructed in assessing proper splint fit, including skin inspection, to prevent the incidence of skin breakdown from excessive pressure. Providing verbal and written instructions is recommended. Additionally, labeling the splint and supplying photos of its proper fit may be helpful.

Regular re-evaluation of splint fit

A splint's effectiveness is only as good as its fit. Burn patients commonly require varying thickness of bandages to cover their wounds under the areas being splinted. Bandage thickness can affect the position of the involved area and can alter optimal fit. As layers of bandage increase, a splint's design must be adjusted to fit correctly.[30] For example, the metacarpophalangeal (MCP) crease of a resting hand splint should be moved proximally as the hand dressing thickness increases.[30] In the later stages of burn rehabilitation, bandage thickness becomes less of an issue and, instead, poor fit can be caused by increased activity or the slick nature of pressure garment material.

As scar tissue lengthens and ROM gains are made, a splint needs to be adjusted to account for these changes. This may include remolding a static splint or changing the angle of pull on a static progressive or dynamic splint. The size of the splint may also have to be altered as changes in edema occur. Strap placement should be re-evaluated as changes in splint position or design are made. Straps provide strategic stabilization and are critical for optimal positioning of involved structures. For example, a forearm-based resting hand splint must have one strap over the dorsal wrist for wrist extension to facilitate tenodesis, one strap over the proximal phalanges to secure MCP flexion, and a third strap on the proximal forearm to stabilize the splint (**Fig. 7**).

Special hand consideration

The hand is one of the most commonly affected sites for developing a burn scar contracture.[1,31–33] The hand is also the most frequently splinted body region after a burn.[16] The superficial nature of tendons and joints in the hand places burn patients at great risk for damage to these structures, causing deformities, such as claw hand deformity, boutonnière, or mallet deformity.[34] A review of a large adult sample of severe hand burns showed that 81% of patients had abnormal ROM if the burns involved the tendons or joints; however, almost 81% had normal or near-normal

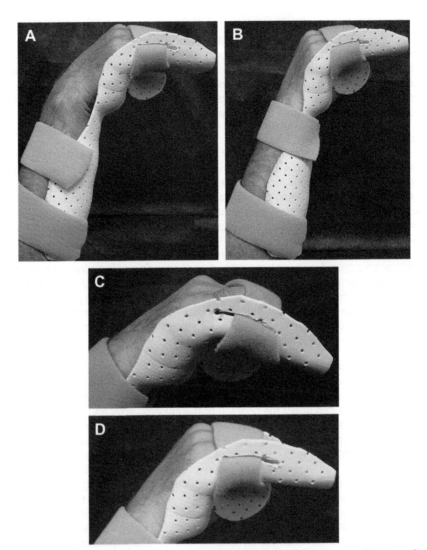

Fig. 7. Effect of strap placement on a resting hand splint. (*A*) Improper wrist strap placement resulting in wrist flexion. (*B*) Proper wrist strap placement providing relative wrist extension. (*C*) Improper digital strap placement facilitating proximal interphalangeal (PIP) flexion and MCP joint flexion. (*D*) Proper digital strap placement over proximal phalanx promoting MCP joint flexion and PIP joint extension.

ROM with deep partial-thickness or full-thickness burns that did not involve tendons or joints.[35] Thus, extreme care should be made with splinting or positioning to protect the soft tissue over joints after a deep partial-thickness or full-thickness burn or after skin grafting. The development of peripheral neuropathies that affect the hand can result in muscle imbalances that can potentially increase the risk of developing deformities as well. Deeply burned hands are commonly splinted in the intrinsic plus position[1] (MCP flexion and IP extension) acutely. This position places the collateral ligaments at the MCP joint in a lengthened or safe position and reduces the stress placed on the superficial tendons of the extensor mechanism over the IP joints. This position also places the hand in the antideformity position as dorsal hand edema promotes wrist flexion, MCP hyperextension, and IP flexion (**Fig. 8**).[36] Consideration must be given, however, to the impact that prolonged positioning in the intrinsic plus position has on contributing to tightness of the intrinsic musculature of the hand. The presence of tightness in these muscles can limit digital ROM and possibly lead to swan-neck deformities.[37] Clinicians should incorporate intrinsic elongation into a patient's exercise program if there are any signs of intrinsic muscle tightness. Palmar burns are routinely placed in finger extension and thumb radial abduction.[8] If both dorsal and palmar burns are present, the clinician must prioritize the desired position based on contracture risk.

Splint fabrication time

A recent study evaluating time demands of burn rehabilitation staff showed that splint fabrication was the most time-consuming task for staff compared with other components of treatment.[38] Splint fabrication is an integral component of burn rehabilitation demanding a significant amount of staff time and, therefore, this must be considered when developing a comprehensive care plan and determining staff ratios.[1]

Splint wearing schedule

The ideal splint wearing schedule has not yet been established.[14] The biomechanical model used in burn rehabilitation[5,39] suggests that the longer a splint is worn, the greater the chance for tissue lengthening. Some practitioners use a 2-hours-on, 2-hours-off wearing protocol[1,14] that may have resulted from a reference advocating such a schedule to prevent splint contamination[40] or from the common positioning schedule of turning patients every 2 hours for optimal pressure relief.[5,41] Some clinicians advocate performing active ROM during the day and splint wear only at night.[1,42] An animal study demonstrated that 6 hours of stress was needed to properly orient developing scar tissue.[20] Regular clinical evaluation of ROM and function is necessary to determine ideal splint wearing schedules for individual patients. Schedules should be determined and adjusted according to the observed changes in passive ROM and activity level.

CASTING

An alternative to splint use is cast application. Cast fabrication is described elsewhere for both the adult and pediatric patient populations.[43–46] Casting has been used as an anticontracture device for the hand,[45–49] wrist,[47,50] elbow,[50,51] axilla,[52] knee,[50] and ankle[50,53] as well as for protection after skin grafting.[44] The reported frequency of cast change ranges from daily to every 10 days.[47,48,50–53] Casting works based on the biomechanic principle of stress relaxation in much the same way as does a static

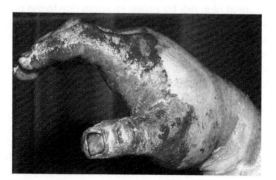

Fig. 8. Edematous hand promotes antideformity position.

splint. One major advantage of casting patients compared with splinting is that a cast is unable to be removed easily. Clinicians need to provide adequate pressure relief over bony prominences, however, to prevent skin breakdown.

BURN REHABILITATION PHASES

Burn rehabilitation is a continuum of care that consists of acute, intermediate, and long-term rehabilitation phases (see **Fig. 1**).[3] The acute phase begins at the time of admission and extends until 50% wound closure is achieved or skin grafting has begun.[3] The intermediate phase constitutes the time surrounding wound closure extending to complete wound closure.[3] The long-term phase starts at wound closure and continues to the period in which the patient has received maximal benefit from rehabilitation to include reconstructive surgery.[3] There is some overlap of these phases dependent on the stage of healing that is taking place for multiple wounds.[3] Clinical priorities change throughout this continuum, and, therefore, the goals of splinting and positioning shift for each phase.

Acute Rehabilitation Phase

Managing edema associated with a burn is a primary rehabilitation goal during the first few days after a burn. Because edema generally peaks within 12 to 48 hours post burn,[8,54,55] it is important to initiate proper positioning on admission. The presence of edema can limit ROM, impair wound healing, and lead to vascular compromise.[8,54] Edema after a burn can affect all parts of the body, including nonburned tissue[55]; thus, elevation of any edematous area is paramount during the acute or resuscitation phase. Elevation is commonly used to facilitate edema reduction. Elevation of the extremities should include the hand or foot being placed above the elbow or knee, which should be at or above heart level.[8,9,56] Although elevation is the primary means of edema control during the acute phase, using a resting hand splint may help oppose the deforming force that edema places on the hand and wrist.[1] Caution is advised, however, with any splint used during the acute phase due to the risk of causing excessive external pressure leading to tissue ischemia.[1] Splint application with constrictive bandages is not recommended during the initial resuscitation phase. Appropriate positioning and splinting can also protect the healing wound, provide pressure relief, and help prevent contractures in the acute phase of rehabilitation.[8] Recent trends have demonstrated an increase in anticontracture positioning and an increased frequency of splint application with both deep partial-thickness burns and full-thickness burns on admission.[15,57]

In the acute rehabilitation phase, positioning and splinting are also used for pressure relief. Burn patients are at high risk for pressure sores due to the presence of multiple factors that can contribute to impaired skin integrity. These include, but are not limited to, open wounds with associated drainage, shear, friction, and potential for unrelieved pressure.[8,58] Areas highly susceptible to skin breakdown are the heels,[55] sacrum, ankles, wrists, elbows, and occipital area.[8] Some options for splinting and positioning devices can be found at burntherapist.com.[59]

Intermediate Rehabilitation Phase

The intermediate rehabilitation phase begins with skin grafting and can include the wound contraction process for nongrafted wounds and ends at wound closure. Positioning and splinting priorities are aimed at protecting skin grafts and facilitating wound healing while maintaining tissue elongation. Managing edema may also still need to be addressed in this phase. Positioning and splinting can be used to prevent maceration of the superficial wound by elevating or suspending the donor site away from bed contact (**Fig. 9**).[60–62] Static splints are the primary type of splint used during the intermediate phase of rehabilitation due to the combined intent to protect skin grafts from shear while maintaining a position required for tissue elongation.

Immobilization after a split-thickness or full-thickness skin graft is a generally accepted practice for skin graft adherence. The use of splints to achieve immobilization is variable, however.[15,17,57] Some clinicians prefer not to splint over a fresh skin graft due to concerns that the splint may cause pressure or shear that may lead to graft failure. Engrav and colleagues[63] demonstrated that the application of splinting devices immediately after skin grafting did not damage grafts of the face and neck. Recent trends show that an increased number of therapists are applying splints after acute skin grafting and supports the notion that splint use for skin graft protection is gaining acceptance.[15,57] The period of immobilization after skin grafting and the method of immobilization vary among clinicians. The immobilization period after skin grafting typically lasts from 3 to 7 days.[1,8] Adequate immobilization can be accomplished by using prefabricated splints, negative pressure wound dressings,[1,8,64] or custom thermoplastic splints. The position of immobilization is dependent on the location of the graft and clinician preference. Surgeons and therapists should discuss desired position and duration of patient immobilization. Although skin graft adherence is the primary objective after skin grafting, the concept of adequate tissue length should also be considered during the procedure. Placing an excised area in a position that requires a greater amount of skin transfer may help reduce ROM loss after surgery due to contraction. Maintenance of this position during the immobilization phase also is beneficial. When possible, having a burn therapist present in the operating room during surgery to assist with adequate positioning is recommended, especially if a negative pressure wound dressing is used to provide immobilization for a hand.[1] A cases series[65] reported a reduced rate of axillary contractures with splint use after skin grafting; however, controlled prospective studies are needed to establish the effectiveness of splinting after skin grafting.[1]

Long-Term Rehabilitation Phase

The long-term rehabilitation phase represents the longest duration of all of the phases. This stage of care spans from the time of wound closure to the point that a plateau is reached with rehabilitation.[3] The rehabilitation emphasis during this phase is to prevent, minimize, and/or correct contractures.[8] Because scar maturation occurs

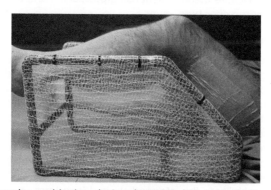

Fig. 9. Lower-extremity positioning device. (*From* Hedman TL, Chapman TT, Dewey WS, et al. Two simple leg net devices designed to protect lower-extremity skin grafts and donor sites and prevent decubitus ulcer. J Burn Care Res 2007;28(1):115–9; with permission.)

throughout this stage of recovery, ROM gains can be achieved with tissue lengthening using the principles of stress relaxation[23] or tissue creep.[8,66,67] Positioning devices and splints provide a means of delivering a desired low-load force for a long duration.[29] The combination of low-load force and long-duration hold provides the preferred stress for scar tissue lengthening. Prompt attention to lengthening scar tissue limits the likelihood that underlying joint capsular tightness or other soft tissue contracture will develop. Static splinting remains highly used during the long-term phase, both after reconstructive surgery and for increasing soft tissue length if an ROM deficit is noted.[15–17] Static progressive and dynamic splints are often used as corrective devices in this phase of recovery. Due to the extended duration of the long-term rehabilitation phase and associated scar maturation, it is common to alternate the use of static, static progressive, and dynamic splints as ROM and surgical needs change. For optimal outcome, the clinician must continue to reassess the effectiveness of a splinting and positioning program while making adjustments and progressions as needed throughout this rehabilitation phase.

SPECIAL CONSIDERATIONS FOR CONTRACTURE MANAGEMENT IN CHILDREN

The basic principles of scar contracture management (discussed previously) apply to patients who have suffered a burn, regardless of their age. Techniques used to apply positioning and splinting principles, however, may be considerably different for children than adults. Children are dynamic human beings who progress through a series of predictable physical, cognitive, emotional, and psychosocial developmental stages.[68] A variety of factors related to a child's development can affect the success of positioning and splinting regimens aimed at preventing, minimizing, or correcting burn scar contracture. Often, young children have not developed the cognitive reasoning to fully comprehend the benefits of such interventions, which leads to increased anxiety and decreased cooperation. Furthermore, a child's small body size, increased activity level, and decreased attention span create challenges with fabrication, fit, and compliance of positioning and splinting devices. Children are physically and emotionally dependent on a larger family unit, so all treatments must incorporate parents, caregivers, or other family members for greatest success. The positioning and splinting goals (described previously) for each stage of burn rehabilitation apply to children as well but with special consideration given to the unique characteristics of developing children. This article describes strategies for improving the effectiveness of contracture management using positioning and splinting techniques specifically with children after burn injury.

Pediatric Positioning Strategies

Developing an effective antideformity positioning program for a young child often proves challenging for a burn therapist. Traditional positioning devices, such as pillows, wedges, bolsters, and linens, which are used with adult patients, may be less effective when used with children due to their elevated activity level and lack of understanding of the importance of compliance. More body-encompassing positioning devices, such as slings and foam/gel positioning devices, may prove effective for positioning to relieve pressure or prevent contractures in the acute rehabilitation stage (**Fig. 10**). Such devices are versatile and accommodate a child's small size while facilitating any developmental needs.

As children gain mobility in the intermediate and long-term rehabilitation phases, positioning devices typically are more successful if the environment is concurrently managed to sustain a child's attention. Providing engaging, age-appropriate, and enjoyable activities improve a child's compliance and cooperation. For example, after contracture release of the anterior neck, when immobilization of the neck in an extended position is required, an inverted television has been used to allow school-aged children to engage in age-appropriate video game play or television viewing and improve cooperation with a prolonged positioning program.[69] Educating caregivers and parents on proper positioning and, when appropriate, involving them in routine monitoring of a child's position can improve overall compliance as well.

When possible, ROM should be maintained with active exercises, function, and play. Positioning programs should be used while a child is at rest. Active ROM has been shown to facilitate functional movement, have positive effects on conditioning, and reduce edema.[13] Active motion also capitalizes on children's natural motivation to move and interact with the environment versus restricting motion, which can increase anxiety or agitation in children. When immobilization is necessary to protect wounds or grafts or when ROM cannot be maintained with active exercises and positioning, however, then passive positioning and splinting devices become necessary.

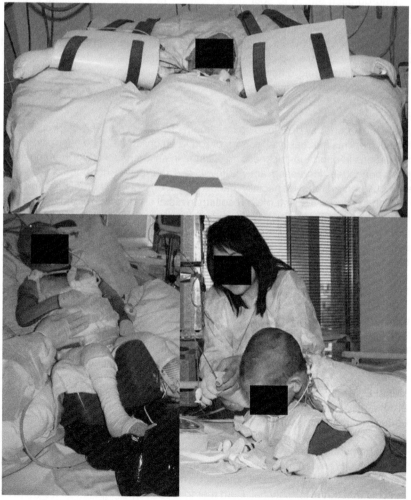

Fig. 10. Pediatric positioning device.

Pediatric Splinting Strategies

Splinting children is not just a matter of reducing the size of an adult splint and donning it. There are special considerations for children in almost every aspect of splint fabrication and use.

Splint design

Choosing the appropriate splint design for a child can be a learning process for a burn therapist. The splint chosen should appropriately fit the smaller limb segments of a child and still meet its intended goals. Dynamic splints, despite showing improvements in ROM in adults,[25] are used less often with small children because they contain small parts and protruding objects, both of which may be unsafe for children.[70] In addition, moveable parts are difficult to anchor to small levers and the cognition and responsibilities needed for proper fit of dynamic splints may be inappropriate for children's cognitive level or difficult for parents to continually monitor.[70] Alternatively, static and static progressive splints are used more often to provide a low-load, long-duration stress to scar tissue. Similar to adults, static splints should be fabricated after SLI and donned with the tissue at a safe maximal length to maintain passive ROM, then remolded or adjusted as changes in motion are achieved. With children, special care should be taken to keep the design simple and low profile and to avoid detachable parts or sharp edges. Pediatric splint designs should also consider other anatomic differences between children and adults, such as thinner, more fragile skin and joint hypermobility.[12]

Splint fit

Even the most perfectly designed splint is ineffective if it is not worn appropriately. As with adults, splints can easily shift, slip, or rotate on children due to fluctuating edema and variations in bandage thickness.[30] Splint fit in children can be further impaired by small appendages, increased activity level, and decreased cooperation. The small size of children's limbs (especially hands and feet) leaves therapists short levers with which to anchor a splint, often resulting in distal slippage or rotation of the splint. If not carefully monitored, this can lead to discomfort, skin breakdown, or exacerbation of a contracture position at a joint. To enhance proper fit, splints should be made with longer levers so that they can be anchored more effectively.[70] Care should be taken, however, to avoid making them so long that baby fat causes pinching with movement at the proximal joint.

Decreased surface area of a small splinted limb reduces the space available for appropriate strapping. Narrowing the straps to fit a splint to a small limb may not be an option in the acute stages of burn recovery due to shifting edema and the risk of constriction. An effective alternative is to use elastic compression bandages or self-adhesive circumferential wraps to encase the entire splint and distribute pressure evenly while securing the splint in place against slipping.[12] Children tend to be more active than adults, more resistant to splint application, and masters at self-removal of splints. By using a proper size self-adhesive circumferential wrap, a splint is better secured in place with movement and or attempts at removal. If a child persists with unwanted doffing of a splint, anti-Houdini options for anchoring splints should be considered.[70] Many splint designs have been established specifically for children with consideration for small body size and increased activity level.[71–74]

Younger children are not always able to fully communicate their needs and concerns regarding splint comfort. Therefore, monitoring the fit of a splint, especially after initial fabrication, is essential. Burn therapists should evaluate splint comfort and fit through careful observation of the child, regular examination of underlying tissue, periodic motor screening, and continual communication with nursing staff and care-givers. Splints should be well labeled and diagrams or photographs provided to nursing staff for proper application and monitoring. When appropriate, parents can be instructed on splint fit and skin inspection. Splints made for use in the intermediate and long-term phases of rehabilitation must continue to be evaluated regularly at follow-up visits and adjusted as necessary for growth or changes in available motion.

Fabrication

Successful fabrication of splints for children with burn injury requires not only technical knowledge of splint mechanics and skilled manipulation of splinting materials but also artful engagement of children. To decrease children's anxiety and encourage cooper-ation, therapists should create a nonthreatening environment, prepare caregivers and children with information about the splint fabrication process, work efficiently, and mold properly on the first attempt. Creating a safe and comfortable physical environ-ment in advance includes having needed equipment within therapist reach and keeping cords and hot pans out of reach of children and sharp instruments out of sight.[75] Introducing the splint material to children, allowing them to touch it, or fabri-cating a small splint on a doll or parent first, works to familiarize children with the splint fabrication process and reduce anxiety.[75,76]

Decreasing children's anxiety helps somewhat to keep them still during splint fabri-cation, but children's decreased attention span or increased pain or sensitivity requires that therapists work quickly and avoid multiple failed attempts.[75] Splint fabri-cation can be done in stages if there are greater time demands for complex splint designs or if the involved areas are sensitive or have limited accessibility. Patterns or photocopies taken of the limb segment can be made in advance to reduce anxiety-provoking treatments and improve patient tolerance. Therapists can use another time-saving technique when fabricating a splint by using the uninvolved extremity or an extremity of a similarly sized sibling to form part of the splint, reserving manipulation of precision areas for the affected side.

Selection of the proper materials for a given patient eases the process of fabrication. Thermoplastic materials used should have high memory, so they can be remolded as edema and bandage thickness changes, yet have stretch and conformability that allows for efficient and precise shaping as needed. Children are especially fearful of warm or hot material; therefore, it may be necessary to let the material cool longer than what is ideal for splint fabrication before placing the material onto a child. Splint-ing over a layer of stockinette can further reduce the amount of heat felt by a child.

A portion of children's willingness to wear a splint is dependent on their perception of the splint. Creating a visually appealing splint and involving a child in the creation process enhance a child's interest and acceptance of wearing a splint. Techniques for making splints more kid friendly are found in **Box 1**. If children show persistent noncompliance and are at risk for contracture development, then serial casting is a treatment option that has shown good outcome with children.[44,53]

Splint wearing schedule

Although the ideal splint wearing schedule for burn patients has yet to be determined, therapists can evaluate the therapeutic benefit of the prescribed splint by monitoring changes in ROM. Decisions regarding frequency and duration of splint wear vary depending on patient needs and situation. In addition to assessment of ROM, pedi-atric burn therapists must consider children's developmental needs, activity level, motivation for movement and play, and scar characteristics when determining an optimal splint wearing schedule.

Box 1
Techniques for making splints kid friendly

- Use colored straps, wraps, and materials
- Allow children to decorate splint and straps with nontoxic colored markers
- Use rub-on tattoos, stickers, or shapes from thermoplastic scraps for decoration
- Round edges
- Avoid small or detachable parts
- Fabricate matching splint for a favorite doll or stuffed animal
- Name the splints to create positive personifications
- Liken the splint to a superhero's gadget or a princess' royal adornment

---

SUMMARY

Whether a patient with burn injury is an adult or child, contracture management should be the primary focus of burn rehabilitation throughout the continuum of care. Positioning and splinting are crucial components of a comprehensive burn rehabilitation program that emphasizes contracture prevention. The emphasis of these devices throughout the phases of rehabilitation fluctuates to meet the changing needs of patients with burn injury. Early, effective, and consistent use of positioning devices and splints is recommended for successful management of burn scar contracture.

REFERENCES

1. Richard R, Baryza M, Carr J, et al. Burn rehabilitation and research: proceedings of a consensus summit. J Burn Care Res 2009;30:543–73.
2. Leblebici B, Adam M, Bağiş S, et al. Quality of life after burn injury: the impact of joint contracture. J Burn Care Res 2006;27:864–8.
3. Richard R, Hedman T, Quick C, et al. A clarion to recommit and reaffirm burn rehabilitation. J Burn Care Res 2008;29:425–32.
4. Ilizarov GA. The tension-stress effect on the genesis and growth of tissues—part I. Clin Orthop Relat Res 1989;238:249–81.
5. Richard R, Steinlage R, Staley M, et al. Mathematic model to estimate change in burn scar length required for joint range of motion. J Burn Care Rehabil 1996;17: 436–43.
6. Richard R, Lester M, Miller S, et al. Identification of cutaneous functional units related to burn scar contracture development. J Burn Care Res 2009;30:625–31.
7. Fung YC. Biomechanics: mechanical properties of living tissues. New York: Springer-Verlag; 1981.
8. Hedman TL, Quick CD, Richard RL, et al. Rehabilitation of burn casualties. In: Lenhart MK, editor. Textbooks of military medicine, care of the combat amputee. Falls Church (VA): Office of the Surgeon General, Department of the Army; 2009. p. 277–380.
9. Apfel L, Irwin C, Staley M, et al. Approaches to positioning the burn patient. In: Richard R, Staley M, editors. Burn care and rehabilitation: principles and practice. Philadelphia: F.A. Davis Company; 1994. p. 221–41.
10. Birch JR, Eakins B, Gosen J, et al. Musculoskeletal management of the severely burned child. Can Med Assoc J 1976;115:533–6.

11. Chapman TT. Burn scar contracture management. J Trauma 2007;62(Suppl 6): S8.
12. Taggart P, Haining R. Rehabilitation of burn injuries. In: Molnar G, Alexander M, editors. Pediatric rehabilitation. 3rd edition. Philadelphia: Hanley & Belfus, Inc; 1999. p. 355–9.
13. Schnebly W, Ward R, Warden G, et al. A nonsplinting approach to the care of the thermally injured patient. J Burn Care Rehabil 1989;10:263–6.
14. Richard R, Ward R. Splinting strategies and controversies. J Burn Care Rehabil 2005;26:392–6.
15. Richard R, Staley M, Miller S, et al. To splint or not to splint-past philosophy and present practice: part I. J Burn Care Rehabil 1996;17:444–53.
16. Richard R, Staley M, Miller S, et al. To splint or not to splint-past philosophy and present practice: part II. J Burn Care Rehabil 1997;18:64–71.
17. Richard R, Staley M, Miller S, et al. To splint or not to splint-past philosophy and present practice: part III. J Burn Care Rehabil 1997;18:251–5.
18. Leman C. Splints and accessories following burn reconstruction. Clin Plast Surg 1992;19:721–31.
19. Linares H, Kischer C, Dobrkovsky M, et al. On the origin of the hypertrophic scar. J Trauma 1973;13:70–5.
20. Arem AJ, Madden JW. Effects of stress on healing wounds: intermittent noncyclical tension. J Surg Res 1976;20:93–102.
21. Huang T, Blackwell S, Lewis S. Ten years of experience in managing patients with burn contractures of axilla, elbow, wrist, and knee joints. Plast Reconstr Surg 1978;61(1):70–6.
22. Bunchman HH II, Huang TT, Larson DL, et al. Prevention and management of contractures in patients with burns of the neck. Am J Surg 1975;130:700–3.
23. Richard R, Miller S, Staley M, et al. Multimodal versus progressive treatment techniques to correct burn scar contractures. J Burn Care Rehabil 2000;21: 506–12.
24. Schultz-Johnson K. Static progressive splinting. J Hand Ther 2002;15:163–78.
25. Richard R, Shanesy CP III, Miller S. Dynamic versus static splints: a prospective case for sustained stress. J Burn Care Rehabil 1995;16:284–7.
26. Flowers KR. A proposed decision heirarchy for splinting the stiff joint, with an emphasis on force application parameters. J Hand Ther 2002;15(2):158–62.
27. Richard R, Johnson R, Miller S. A compendium of customized burn splint designs. J Burn Care Rehabil 2003;24:S142.
28. Richard R, Chapman T, Dougherty M, et al. An atlas and compendium of burn splints. San Antonio (TX): Reg Richard, Inc; 2005.
29. Fess EE. Principles and methods of splinting for mobilization of joints. In: Mackin EJ, Callahan AD, Skirven TM, et al, editors. Rehabilitation of the hand and upper extremity. 5th edition. St. Louis (MO): Mosby, Inc; 2002. p. 1818–27.
30. Richard R, Schall S, Staley M, et al. Hand burn splint fabrication: correction for bandage thickness. J Burn Care Rehabil 1994;15:369–71.
31. Dobbs E, Curreri P. Burns: analysis of results of physical therapy in 681 patients. J Trauma 1972;12:242–8.
32. Kraemer M, Jones T, Deitch E. Burn contractures: incidence, predisposing factors, and results of surgical therapy. J Burn Care Rehabil 1988;9:261–5.
33. Schneider J, Holavanahalli R, Helm P, et al. Contractures in burn injury part 2: investigating joints of the hand. J Burn Care Res 2008;29:606–13.
34. Esselman P, Thombs B, Magyar-Russell G, et al. Burn rehabilitation: state of the science. Am J Phys Med Rehabil 2006;85:383–413.

35. Sheridan R, Hurley J, Smith M, et al. The acutely burned hand: management and outcome based on a ten-year experience with 1047 acute hand burns. J Trauma 1995;38:406–11.

36. Madden J, Enna C. The management of acute thermal injuries to the upper extremity. J Hand Surg Am 1983;8:785–8.

37. Rosenthal EA. The extensor tendons: anatomy and management. In: Mackin EJ, Callahan AD, Skirven TM, et al, editors. Rehabilitation of the hand and upper extremity. 5th edition. St. Louis (MO): Mosby, Inc; 2002. p. 498–541.

38. Dewey WS, Richard RL, Casey JC, et al. Burn rehabilitation time study. J Burn Care Res 2009;30(2):S137.

39. Richard R. Burns. In: Jacobs ML, Austin N, editors. Splinting the hand and upper extremity: principles and process. Baltimore (MD): Lippincott Williams & Wilkens; 2003. p. 446–55.

40. Malick MH. Management of the severely burned patient. Br J Occup Ther 1975; 38:76–80.

41. Salcido R. Patient turning schedules: why and how often? Adv Skin Wound Care 2004;17:156.

42. Helm PA, Kevorkian CG, Lushbaugh M, et al. Burn injury: rehabilitation management in 1982. Arch Phys Med Rehabil 1982;63:6–16.

43. Staley M, Serghiou M. Casting guidelines, tips, and techniques: proceedings from the 1997 American Burn Association PT/OT casting workshop. J Burn Care Rehabil 1998;19:254–60.

44. Ricks NR, Meagher DP. The benefits of plaster casting for lower-extremity burns after grafting in children. J Burn Care Rehabil 1992;13:465–8.

45. Jackson RD. The MCP block cast with flexion glove: an alternative method over traditional splinting. J Burn Care Rehabil 1997;18:S175.

46. Flesch P. Casting the young and the restless. Proc Am Burn Assoc 1985;17:120.

47. Walker K, Serghiou M, Duplantis C, et al. Serial casting with silicone for volar hand/wrist contractures. J Burn Care Rehabil 1997;18:S173.

48. Harris LD, Hatler B, Adams S, et al. Serial casting and its efficacy in the treatment of the burned hand. Proc Am Burn Assoc 1993;25:129.

49. Torres-Gray D, Johnson J, Greenspan B, et al. The fabrication and use of the removable digit casts to improve range of motion at the proximal interphalangeal joint. Proc Am Burn Assoc 1993;25:217.

50. Bennett GB, Helm P, Purdue GF, et al. Serial casting: a method for treating burn contractures. J Burn Care Rehabil 1989;10:543–5.

51. Cattanach LB, Rivers E, Solem L, et al. Achieving optimal elbow extension using the serial, "fall-out" elbow cast. Proc Am Burn Assoc 1990;22:138.

52. Kirby J, Facchine SL, Slater H, et al. Serial casting for axilla contractures. Proc Am Burn Assoc 1992;24:11.

53. Ridgway CL, Daugherty MB, Warden GD. Serial casting as a technique to correct burn scar contractures, a case report. J Burn Care Rehabil 1992;12: 67–72.

54. Kramer G, Lund T, Herndon D. Pathophysiology of burn shock and burn edema. In: Herndon DN, editor. Total burn care. 2nd edition. New York: WB Saunders; 2002. p. 78–87.

55. Demling RH. The burn edema process: current concepts. J Burn Care Rehabil 2005;26:207–27.

56. Hildebrant W, Herrmann J, Stegemann J. Vascular adjustment and fluid absorption in the human forearm during elevation. Eur J Appl Physiol Occup Physiol 1993;66:397–400.

57. Whitehead C, Serghiou M. A 12-year comparison of common therapeutic interventions in the burn unit. J Burn Care Res 2009;30:281–7.
58. Gordon MD, Gottschlich MM, Hevlig EI, et al. Review of evidence-based practice for the prevention of pressure sores in burn patients. J Burn Care Rehabil 2004; 25(5):388–410.
59. Available at: www.burntherapist.com. Accessed March 9, 2011.
60. Hedman TL, Chapman TT, Dewey WS, et al. Two simple leg net devices designed to protect lower-extremity skin grafts and donor sites and prevent decubitus ulcer. J Burn Care Res 2007;28(1):115–9.
61. Serghiou M, Farmer S, Rubio M, et al. A suspension device to protect delicate grafts on extremities and prevent pressure sores during immobilization. J Burn Care Rehabil 2005;26:S165.
62. Salinas RD, Hedman TL, Quick CD, et al. Ventilation back ramp designed to prevent suppurative donor sites and accelerate healing time. J Burn Care Res 2007;28:S109.
63. Engrav L, Macdonald L, Covey M, et al. Do splinting and pressure devices damage new grafts? (appliances and new grafts). J Burn Care Rehabil 1983;4: 107–8.
64. Mendez-Eastman S. Guidelines for using negative pressure wound therapy. Adv Skin Wound Care 2001;14:314–22.
65. Vehmeyer-Heeman M, Lommers B, Van den Kerckhove E, et al. Axillary burns: extended grafting and early splinting prevents contractures. J Burn Care Rehabil 2005;26:539–42.
66. Escoffier C, de Rigal J, Rochefort A, et al. Age-related mechanical properties of human skin: an in vivo study. J Invest Dermatol 1989;93(3):353–7.
67. Wilhelmi BJ, Blackwell SJ, Mancoll JS, et al. Creep vs stretch: a review of the viscoelastic properties of skin. Ann Plast Surg 1998;41(2):215–9.
68. Sroufe LA, Cooper RG, DeHart GB. Child development, its nature and course. 2nd edition. New York (NY): McGraw-Hill, Inc; 1992.
69. Hurlin Foley K, Kaulkin C, Palmieri T, et al. Inverted television and video games to maintain neck extension. J Burn Care Rehabil 2001;22:366–8.
70. Hogan L, Udisky T. Pediatric splinting, selection, fabrication, and clinical application of upper extremity splints. San Antonio (TX): Therapy Skill Builders; 1998.
71. Malick MH, Carr JA, editors. Manual on management of the burn patient. Pittsburgh (PA): Harmarville Rehabilitation Center; 1982. p. 60.
72. Kaufman T, Newman RA, Weinberg A, et al. The Kerlix tongue-depressor splint for skin-grafted areas in burned children. J Burn Care Rehabil 1989;10:462–3.
73. Ward RS, Schnebly A, Kravitz M, et al. Have you tried the sandwich splint? A method of preventing hand deformities in children. J Burn Care Rehabil 1989; 10:83–5.
74. Schwanholt C, Daugherty MB, Gaboury T, et al. Splinting the pediatric palmar burn. J Burn Care Rehabil 1992;13:460–4.
75. Wilton J. Hand splinting principles of design and fabrication. London: WB Saunders Company Ltd; 1997. p. 15–7.
76. Daugherty MB, Carr-Collins JA. Splinting techniques for the burn patient. In: Richard R, Staley M, editors. Burn care and rehabilitation: principles and practice. Philadelphia: F.A. Davis Company; 1994. p. 284–5.

Hand Burns

Karen J. Kowalske, MD

KEYWORDS

• Hand burns • Contracture • Rehabilitation • Outcomes

Burn rehabilitation cannot be reviewed without a significant focus on the hand. Although the surface area of the hand is only 3%, the functional consequences are so impairing that any 2nd or 3rd degree hand burn is classified as a major burn injury, and referral to a burn center is recommended.[1] Also, most individuals with large burns have some involvement of the hand.[2] Contracture is a common complication following hand burns,[3] and limitations in the hand result in significant functional limitations and decrease in quality of life.[4,5] A comprehensive team approach from initial evaluation through long-term follow up is essential to maximize the functional outcome in this population. This team must work together to address wound closure edema, scar contracture, joint deformity, and functional issues.[6]

ACUTE MANAGEMENT

Close evaluation and management of the hand must be done in the very early stages following a burn injury. The surgical evaluation includes overall burn size and total body surface area (TBSA) to facilitate appropriate resuscitation. The hand-specific assessment must include a thorough evaluation of depth of burn. This is particularly important across the dorsal aspect of the digits to assess the risk of tendon exposure or rupture of the extensor mechanism. A neurologic examination should be performed for all patients, but particular attention should be paid in those with circumferential burns or electrical injuries.

With the acute resuscitation there is significant fluid extravasation and associated edema[7] that can lead to a claw hand deformity with hyperextension of the metacarpal phalangeal (MP) and flexion of proximal interphalangeal (PIP).[8] Therefore the initial positioning should be in the antideformity position, which will also help control expanding edema. This is usually done with a classic volar positioning (VPS) splint (**Fig. 1**). If the patient is unable to perform any active exercise, the splint is removed for range of motion with the therapist and for wound care but left in place the rest of the time. Once the patient is alert enough to begin actively using the hand, the splint

This work was supported by funds from the National Institute on Disability and Rehabilitation Research in the Office of Special Education and Rehabilitative Services in the US Department of Education.
Department of Physical Medicine and Rehabilitation, University of Texas SW Medical Center, 5323 Harry Hines Boulevard, Dallas, TX 75390-9055, USA
E-mail address: karen.kowalske@utsouthwestern.edu

Phys Med Rehabil Clin N Am 22 (2011) 249–259
doi:10.1016/j.pmr.2011.03.003
1047-9651/11/$ – see front matter © 2011 Elsevier Inc. All rights reserved.

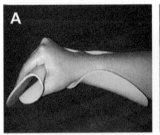
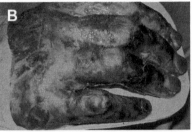

Fig. 1. Volar positioning splint (VPS) used primarily for edema control following an acute burn (A, B).

can be used just at night. The MP hyperextension posture seen in a claw hand deformity is similar to the intrinsic minus hand associated with median and ulnar neuropathy. Differentiating between these two conditions is important, because the treatment approach is very different (**Fig. 2**).

Positioning for those with hand burns is designed to keep MP flexion range of motion, prevent extensor mechanism rupture with PIP and distal interphalangeal (DIP) extension, and help control edema. Elevation of the hand is also helpful to limit edema. Splinting initially is primarily the use of the VPS as outlined previously. Once the wound is mostly closed, alternative splinting to maximize function should be prescribed.

Passive range of motion should begin following initial assessment and advanced to active assistive and active range of motion as the patient is more able to participate. If the burn appears to be deep full thickness, one must be aware of possible disruption of the extensor mechanism either by direct thermal injury or by ischemia.[9] The extent of this injury is difficult to assess with overlying eschar.[10] Therefore all full thickness hand burns should be treated as if the extensor mechanism is jeopardized. Range of motion can be continued using the tendon glide technique. This technique involves mobilizing a single joint while keeping the other joints in extension (ie, flexing the MP while keeping the PIP and DIP in extension, flexing the PIP with the MP and DIP in extension, or flexing the DIP with the MP and PIP in extension). This technique allows for some tendon sliding to decrease the risk of adhesion formation. The tendon should be kept moist, and combined flexion must be absolutely avoided, as this full fisting

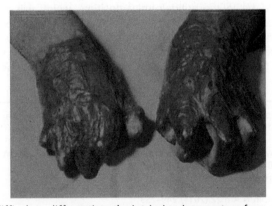

Fig. 2. It is very difficult to differentiate the intrinsic minus posture from neuropathy versus edema.

position can rupture the fragile extensor mechanism. Splinting allows removal for wound care but risks jeopardizing the tendon with patient movement when the splint is not in place. Finger casting leaving the DIP free allows for tendon glide stretching within the cast and provides protection from combined flexion (**Fig. 3**). The downfall of this technique is that the cylindrical nature of the digit makes it difficult to keep the cast in place. Pinning is the most stable solution but may result in digit fusion, particularly if the pin is left in place for more than a few weeks. If the tendon is irreversibly ruptured and fusion is the goal, then the digit should be pinned in a functional position with the PIP in 30° of flexion and DIP in full extension. In these cases, aggressive range of the MP joint to regain flexion is essential for maximizing function.

Superficial or midpartial thickness hand burns heal spontaneously with little cosmetic or functional sequelea.[11] This depth of burn usually does not require hospitalization. Also, isolated unilateral full-thickness hand burns can be managed on an outpatient basis until the time of surgery. For those with bilateral hand burns, hospitalization is usually recommended because of the difficulty of maintaining self-care independence with both hands in dressings. Also, earlier surgery allows the individual to regain functional independence sooner.

Early excision and grafting are the standard of care for treatment of full-thickness hand burns,[8,12–14] but the definition of what is early continues to be debated. Obviously, wound closure decreases edema and helps maximize function, but this cannot be done at the expense of closing larger surfaces in an individual with a very large burn. Using a tourniquet at the time of excision limits blood loss. Tourniquet time and pressure should be monitored closely to avoid underlying tissue or neurologic injury. Full-thickness or split-thickness sheet grafting is recommended to maximize

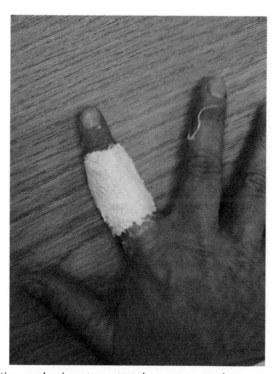

Fig. 3. Finger casting can be done to protect the extensor tendon.

cosmetic and functional outcomes (**Fig. 4**).[15] If the extensor mechanism is exposed, it is likely that the graft will not take over this area. Traditional grafting followed by wound care often results in tendon adherence to the zone that healed by secondary intention. The use of an artificial dermal matrix can help prevent this but requires two surgical procedures, which may not be feasible for those with large burns. Digit amputation is required when the underlying tissue and bone are mummified. Other than in cases of high-voltage electrical injury, amputation is rarely emergent, and delays may help in maximizing length.

OUTPATIENT CARE

Following hospital discharge, the rehabilitation program continues to address many of the ongoing issues associated with hand burns. Despite wound closure, persistent edema may continue to be problematic. Use of an off-the-shelf pressure glove combined with elevation may provide some relief. If the edema persists, an elastic pressure dressing can be used. This is an excellent way to decrease edema but may temporarily limit digit flexion (**Fig. 5**).[16] Custom gloves are a more long-term solution but are expensive and also interfere with functional tasks.[17] A very small percentage of patients with edema develops a syndrome that resembles complex regional pain syndrome (CRPS) type 1. This is mostly seen in patients with partial-thickness burns who do not exercise and develop significant edema. This condition responds to oral steroids and range of motion with full resolution (**Fig. 6**).

Range of motion continues to be an essential component of treatment and recovery. Active assistive range with sustained stretch at or near the point of skin blanching forces the skin cells to divide and lengthen. In general, 20 minutes in the sustained

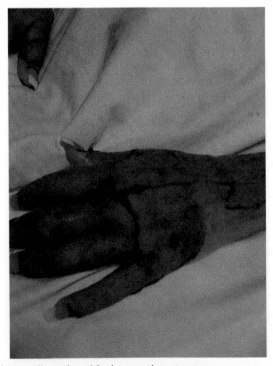

Fig. 4. Sheet grafting will produce ideal cosmetic outcome.

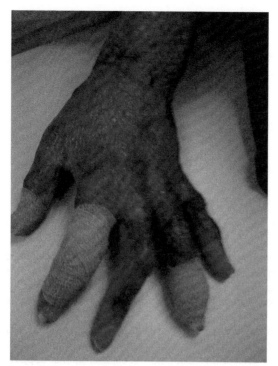

Fig. 5. Elastic dressings to decrease edema.

stretch position is recommended. Moisturizing before stretch decreases the risk of skin tears. Paraffin at 120°F moisturizes and can facilitate relaxation but does not necessarily increase the range of motion gains obtained with stretching alone. Although ultrasound has been recommended by some, there are no definitive studies showing it aides in improving hand range of motion after burn.[6]

Splinting continues to be an adjuvant technique for maintaining scar stretch. The traditional VPS, which is the mainstay during hospitalization, is almost never the splint of choice for an outpatient. Flexion glove with or without an MP block is used to facilitate combined flexion (**Fig. 7**). A palmer conformer is used for facilitating palmer abduction. Ulnar gutter is used to keep the fifth digit from drifting into abduction. Casting has the advantage and disadvantage of being nonremovable. It can give a better stretch for palmer tightness and facilitates compliance particularly in children.

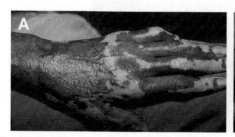
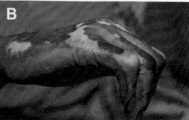

Fig. 6. (*A, B*) Complex regional pain syndrome with edema and decreased finger flexion.

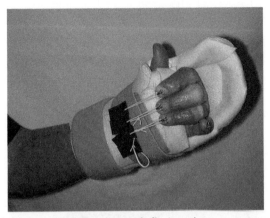

Fig. 7. Metacarpal phalangeal block splint with flexion glove.

Exercise and functional activities are very important components of treatment after hand burn. Strengthening can be done with putty, claw, weights, or activity simulation (**Fig. 8**). Obtaining range of motion and doing activities as before injury is ideal, but when this is not possible, adaptive techniques should be taught to facilitate functional independence.

The hand has many common deformities, including web space contractures; fifth finger abduction deformity; metacarpophalangeal (MCP) joint extension deformities; boutonnière, swan neck and mallet deformities; and palmer cupping.[18] Contractures of the web spaces are common challenges following hand burn. First web space tightness is managed by conformer splinting with the thumb in radial abduction (**Fig. 9**). The other webs are addressed by using elastomer or silicone conformers with counter pressure in the space between the digits (**Fig. 10**). MCP extension deformities are treated with MP blocking splints or casting. The Boutonniere deformity occurs from rupture of the extensor hood at the PIP with volar migration of the central slips. This results in flexion of the PIP and hyperextension of the DIP. Ideally this would be prevented during the acute management, but if it does occur, hand function can be maintained by focusing on MP flexion, allowing the patient to achieve functional grasps (**Fig. 11**). Although Boutonniere deformity can be corrected after traumatic injury, this is very difficult in the burned hand, because the integrity of the dorsal skin is marginal at best. Additionally, the tendon is usually contracted and scarred down.

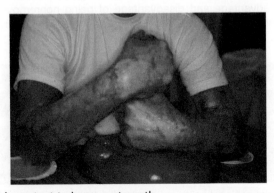

Fig. 8. Exercise is important to improve strength.

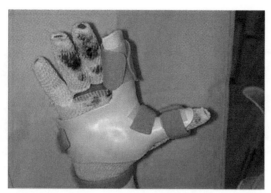

Fig. 9. Splinting provides counter pressure to maintain the first web space.

Swan neck deformity occurs as a result of lateral scar tissue and is difficult to fully correct. Mallet deformity can be partially corrected with splinting, casting, or pinning. Palmer cupping primarily occurs in children with hot contact burns to the palm (**Fig. 12**). With partial thickness palm burns, a palmer conforming splint may hold the palm contour. Unfortunately, children have a tendency to pull the palm into adduction, and the short lever arm makes it difficult to get a good purchase for maintaining stretch within the splint. Therefore, casting may be the best approach. Of note, children less than age 2 have very little wrist contour, which makes it possible for them to pull their arm out of a short arm cast. If positioning is essential, then a long arm cast with the elbow flexed at 90° may be required.

Neuropathy is seen in 12% to 15% of patients with burn injury,[19] and the median and ulnar nerves are often involved.[20] The underlying mechanism of this neuropathy is not known but is presumed to be some form of ischemia, either microvascular from edema, or due to a central immunologic microvascular response. Although electrodiagnostic testing can be performed, it often is not necessary, as the prognosis for recovery is generally good.[20]

Long-term functional outcome is a related to several factors, including depth of burn, edema during the acute period, formation of hypertrophic scar, joint contracture, lack of compliance with therapy regimen, pain, and neuropathy. Superficial and midpartial thickness hand burns heal spontaneously with little to no cosmetic or functional impairment.[11] Deep partial thickness hand burns may heal without grafting but result in significant functional impairment.[11] Therefore, it is recommended that deep partial and full-thickness hand burns be grafted as soon as safely feasible. Unfortunately,

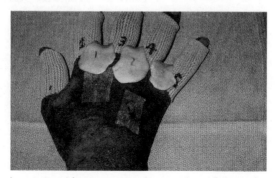

Fig. 10. Elastomer inserts provide pressure to decrease loss of the web spaces.

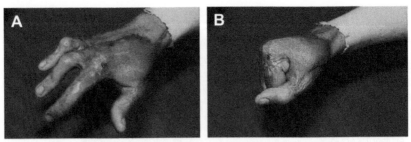

Fig. 11. Boutonniere deformity. Able to fully fist if metacarpal phalangeal flexion is retained (*A, B*).

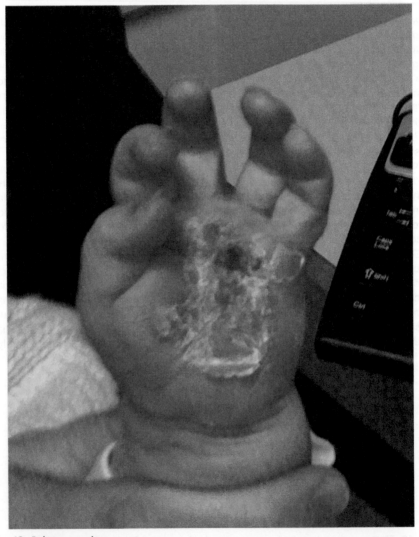

Fig. 12. Palmer cupping.

among those with joint capsule, bone, and extensor mechanism injuries, hand function almost never returns to normal, with persistent loss of range of motion, strength, and dexterity. Despite these limitations, most do regain independence with activities of daily living (ADL).[11]

RANGE OF MOTION AND STRENGTH

The hands represent the most common location of loss of range of motion in patients with burn injury, with the most common contractures being wrist extension and flexion, digit MP flexion, and index finger (PIP) flexion. Study of hand range-of-motion outcomes is very difficult because of the large volume of data (301 measurements per hand) generated. This issue is not easily overcome. To help with dealing with this volume of data, several investigators have used total active motion (TAM).[21,22] This technique adds the flexion and extension range with a loss of full range used as a negative number, giving a normal TAM of 260° for each finger. Although using TAM simplifies the statistics for study individuals with complex loss of range of motion of the hand, this method certainly falls short in truly describing the outcomes. The main challenge of this method is that lacking 20° of extension at the MP is not equivalent to having only 70° of flexion at the MP, yet in the TAM methodology these two are evaluated as equivalent.[23,24]

Patient satisfaction with hand function after burn injury correlates with work performance, aesthetics, pain, and ADLs. It is clear that most patients are satisfied with their outcome, but most have some functional limitations at hospital discharge. Using the Jebsen Hand Test[25] to study individuals with deep full-thickness hand burns showed scores worse than the norms, with the most significant difficulty seen in writing a sentence. Women do better with writing, turning cards, and picking up small objects. Men do better than women on lifting a heavy can. This is likely related to women using their fingernails, which helps with manipulating small objects, and men using their larger hand span, allowing them to lift the heavy can.[23]

The American Medical Association (AMA) has issued guidelines for the assessment of impairment. These guidelines are used to evaluate limitations in strength and range of motion, as well as skin changes. One study of the guidelines showed impairment after major burn injury to be 17% to 20%.[19] Although hand impairment was not selected individually, almost half of the impairment was due to impairment of upper extremity function. In the guidelines, the hands represent 60% of the upper extremity, so it is likely that a significant portion of this impairment was due to limitations in hand function. Community integration and return to work are effected by having a hand burn. Studies have shown mixed results on the effects of hand burn on return to work.[26] The largest of these studies did show that having a hand burn influenced return to work, with those with an arm burn being 73% less likely to return to work at 6 months.[27] Therefore, further evaluation of the effect of hand burn on return to work needs to be conducted.

Like other rehabilitation topics, many areas of burn care are have not been thoroughly evaluated scientifically. A national research forum outlined the following as the top priorities for research in rehabilitation following hand burns[28]:

Determining the best approach to management of the deep hand burn with exposed tendon
Determining the role and benefit of skin substitutes in the management of hand burns
Determining the optimal surgical approach to prevent and treat web space contractures

Determining the optimal timing and components of burn hand therapy, including exercises and modalities

Examining the factors that influence the outcome of partial-thickness hand burns

These questions must be answered in a scientific way to help maximize outcomes while limiting recovery time and overall costs.

In conclusion, hand burns are common and have significant functional consequences. Close attention to edema control and protection of the extensor tendon acutely followed by range of motion, functional training, and splinting and casting as appropriate can maximize functional outcome from this devastating injury.

REFERENCES

1. Available at: http://ameriburn.org/BurnCenterReferralCriteria.pdf. Accessed March 4, 2011.
2. Smith MA, Munster AM, Spence RJ. Burns of the hand and upper limb—a review. Burns 1998;24:493–505.
3. Schneider JC, Holavanahalli R, Helm P, et al. Contractures in burn injury part II: investigating joints of the hand. J Burn Care Res 2008;29:606–13.
4. Baker RA, Jones S, Sanders C, et al. Degree of burn, location of burn, and length of hospital stay as predictors of psychosocial status and physical functioning. J Burn Care Rehabil 1996;17:327–33.
5. Anzarut A, Chen M, Shankowsky H, et al. Quality-of-life and outcome predictors following massive burn injury. Plast Reconstr Surg 2005;116:791–7.
6. Moore ML, Dewey WS, Richard RL. Rehabilitation of the burned hand. Hand Clin 2009;25:529–41.
7. Witte CL, Witte MH, Dumont AE. Significance of protein in edema fluids. Lymphology 1971;4:29–31.
8. Salisbury RE, Wright P. Evaluation of early excision of dorsal burns of the hand. Plast Reconstr Surg 1982;69:670–5.
9. Maisels DO. The middle slip or boutonniere deformity in burned hands. Br J Plast Surg 1965;18:117–29.
10. Hunt JL, Sato RM. Early excision of full-thickness hand and digit burns: factors affecting morbidity. J Trauma 1982;22:414–9.
11. Sheridan RL, Hurley J, Smith MA, et al. The acutely burned hand: management and outcome based on a ten-year experience with 1047 acute hand burns. J Trauma 1995;38:406–11.
12. Burke JF, Bondoc CC, Quinby WC Jr, et al. Primary surgical management of the deeply burned hand. J Trauma 1976;16:593–8.
13. Frist W, Ackroyd F, Burke J, et al. Long-term functional results of selective treatment of hand burns. Am J Surg 1985;149:516–21.
14. van Zuijlen PP, Kreis RW, Vloemans AF, et al. The prognostic factors regarding long-term functional outcome of full-thickness hand burns. Burns 1999;25:709–14.
15. Sterling J, Gibran NS, Klein MB. Acute management of hand burns. Hand Clin 2009;25:453–9.
16. Lowell M, Pirc P, Ward RS, et al. Effect of 3M Coban Self-Adherent Wraps on edema and function of the burned hand: a case study. J Burn Care Rehabil 2003;24:253–8 [discussion: 2].
17. O'Brien KA, Weinstock-Zlotnick G, Sanchez J, et al. Comparison of positive pressure gloves on hand use in uninjured persons. J Burn Care Rehabil 2005;26:363–8 [discussion: 2].

18. Salisbury RE. Reconstruction of the burned hand. Clin Plast Surg 2000;27:65–9.
19. Kowalske K, Holavanahalli R, Helm P. Neuropathy after burn injury. J Burn Care Rehabil 2001;22:353–7 [discussion: 2].
20. Gabriel V, Kowalske KJ, Holavanahalli RK. Assessment of recovery from burn-related neuropathy by electrodiagnostic testing. J Burn Care Res 2009;30: 668–74.
21. Cartotto R. The burned hand: optimizing long-term outcomes with a standardized approach to acute and subacute care. Clin Plast Surg 2005;32:515–27.
22. Harvey KD, Barillo DJ, Hobbs CL, et al. Computer-assisted evaluation of hand and arm function after thermal injury. J Burn Care Rehabil 1996;17:176–80 [discussion: 5].
23. Holavanahalli RK, Helm PA, Gorman AR, et al. Outcomes after deep full-thickness hand burns. Arch Phys Med Rehabil 2007;88:S30–5.
24. Kowalske K. Outcome assessment after hand burns. Hand Clin 2009;25:557–61.
25. Jebsen RH, Taylor N, Trieschmann RB, et al. An objective and standardized test of hand function. Arch Phys Med Rehabil 1969;50:311–9.
26. Hwang YF, Chen-Sea MJ, Chen CL. Factors related to return to work and job modification after a hand burn. J Burn Care Res 2009;30:661–7.
27. Brych SB, Engrav LH, Rivara FP, et al. Time off work and return to work rates after burns: systematic review of the literature and a large two-center series. J Burn Care Rehabil 2001;22:401–5.
28. Kowalske KJ, Greenhalgh DG, Ward SR. Hand burns. J Burn Care Res 2007;28: 607–10.

Neurologic and Musculoskeletal Complications of Burn Injuries

Jeffery C. Schneider, MD[a],*, Huaguang David Qu, MD, MS[a]

KEYWORDS

- Neurologic • Musculoskeletal • Complications • Thermal injury
- Electrical injury

Approximately one-half million people seek medical care for burn injuries each year, including 40,000 hospitalizations, 25,000 admissions to specialized burn centers, and 4000 deaths.[1] With advances in acute management of burns over the past few decades more people are surviving severe burn injuries.[2] As a result, providers are increasingly focused on the long-term management of burn survivors.

Burns are complex injuries that affect almost every organ system of the body and result in numerous long-term complications. Common complications of burn injuries include neurologic and musculoskeletal problems. These complications may develop a few weeks to years after injury, and significantly affects quality of life. Successful management of these complications directly impacts the burn survivor's functional recovery.

The authors address burn-related neurologic and musculoskeletal complications in this article. In addition, electrical burn injuries are discussed because they are a subcategory of burns with significant neurologic and musculoskeletal complications.

NEUROLOGIC INJURIES

Clinically, neurologic complications are often underreported in the literature because the diagnosis is commonly delayed or missed entirely. The neurologic assessment is marred by the complexity of medical problems and impaired consciousness of patients who are critically ill. However, neurologic injuries cause serious debility and functional deficits that impact recovery. Both prevention and identification of neuropathies is an important aspect of burn rehabilitation. The neurologic complications of burn injuries are outlined in **Table 1**.

[a] Department of Physical Medicine and Rehabilitation, Harvard Medical School, Spaulding Rehabilitation Hospital, 125 Nashua Street, Boston, MA 02114, USA
* Corresponding author.
E-mail address: jcschneider@partners.org

Phys Med Rehabil Clin N Am 22 (2011) 261–275
doi:10.1016/j.pmr.2011.01.003
1047-9651/11/$ – see front matter © 2011 Elsevier Inc. All rights reserved.

Table 1
Neurologic complications of burn injuries

Complication	Comments
Mononeuropathy	Length of ICU stay, alcohol, electrical injury, age, and diabetes are risk factors. Specific positions predispose one to compression neuropathy.
Peripheral Polyneuropathy	Length of ICU stay and age are risk factors.
Mononeuritis Multiplex	Not well understood; lower-extremity injuries have better prognosis than upper-extremity injuries.
Pruritus	High incidence; managed with topical and oral medications

Localized Neuropathies

Localized neuropathies are common after burn injuries with an incidence of 15% to 37%.[3,4] Kowalske and colleagues[5] examined 572 burn survivors and found that electrical injury, history of alcohol abuse, and length of intensive-care-unit (ICU) stay are significant risk factors for the development of mononeuropathies. Premorbid factors, such as elderly age and diabetes, are risk factors for the development of peripheral nerve compromise.[4,6] In addition, prevention of compression neuropathy is an important tenet of rehabilitation. Bulky dressings can cause compression to superficial peripheral nerves, and improper and prolonged positioning can cause excessive stretch of nerves. Thus, proper positioning of patients as well as careful monitoring of wound care can mitigate neurologic complications. Clinical pearls of specific mononeuropathies and brachial plexopathy are reviewed in **Table 2**.

In general, poor positioning at the neck and shoulder leads to excessive stretch of the brachial plexus and places the plexus at risk for injury. Also, several bed and intraoperative positions commonly used in the treatment of burn injuries put the plexus at risk. Positioning of the shoulder during grafting of the axilla or lateral chest wall, with abduction of at least 90° and external rotation, places excessive stretch on the plexus.[7] Patients are also placed in this position for alleviation of arm edema and prevention of axillary contractures. An alternate position that does not compromise the brachial plexus involves lying supine with the shoulder in 90° of abduction along with 30° of shoulder horizontal adduction.[7]

Table 2
Localized neuropathies and associated risk factors

Neuropathy	Risk Factors
Brachial plexus	Shoulder abduction >90, external rotation Axilla/lateral chest wall grafting position
Ulnar nerve	Elbow flexion 90°, pronation, tourniquet paralysis
Radial nerve	At spiral groove: resting on side rails, hanging over edge of operating table, tourniquet paralysis At wrist: wrist restraints
Median nerve	Edema, prolonged or repeated wrist hyperextension, tourniquet paralysis
Peroneal nerve	Frog-leg position, lateral decubitus position, metal stirrups, leg straps, bulky dressings
Femoral nerve	Hematoma at femoral triangle, retroperitoneal bleed

In the upper extremity, the ulnar, median, and radial nerves are common sites for development of mononeuropathies. Positioning the elbow in flexion and pronation stretches the ulnar nerve and places it at risk for compression at the cubital tunnel. Median nerve injuries most commonly occur at the wrist. Local edema and prolonged or repeated hyperextension of the wrist compresses the nerve at the carpal tunnel. Clinicians should exercise caution when using wrist splints or an exercise program that includes hyperextension of the wrist. Radial nerve injuries most commonly result from compression at the spiral groove of the humerus. Therefore, arm positions that place the radial nerve at risk for injury include resting it on the bed siderails or hanging it over the edge of the operating table during interventional procedures. In addition, a pure sensory neuropathy results from compression of the superficial cutaneous branch of the radial nerve at the wrist, as with use of wrist restraints. Also, pneumatic tourniquets that are used in the operating room to establish a bloodless field may cause upper-extremity neuropathies. Improper inflation pressures can cause a direct pressure injury of the peripheral nerve at the cuff edge.[8] The radial nerve is most vulnerable, but ulnar and median nerves are also at risk. Mononeuropathies of the upper extremities can also develop as a late complication of heterotopic bone formation. The elbow in particular is a common site of heterotopic ossification (HO) formation thus putting the ulnar nerve at risk.

In the lower extremities, the peroneal and femoral nerves are the most common mononeuropathies. The anatomic course of the peroneal nerve places it at risk with several common positions. Stretch injuries may occur with the frog-leg position, defined as externally rotated and flexed hip, flexed knee, and inverted foot. This position is used by patients with a tender medial thigh or perineal burns and when the bed is short for the patients' height. Compression of the peroneal nerve at the fibular head is common, usually associated with the use of metal stirrups, leg straps, and the lateral decubitus position. Windowing of the dressing over the fibular head, used to relieve pressure, can also cause compression of the peroneal nerve. The femoral nerve is affected less often. Neuropathies develop in the femoral triangle typically because of compression by hematoma from venous or arterial blood draws. The discovery of a femoral nerve injury in patients on anticoagulation or with recent abdominal surgery raises suspicion of a retroperitoneal hemorrhage.[9]

Peripheral Polyneuropathy

The pathophysiology of peripheral neuropathy in burns is complicated and thought to be caused by a combination of direct thermal injury on the nerves, circulating neurotoxins, and changes in distribution of fluid and electrolytes.[10] These factors result from the body's systemic response to the burn injury. After burn injury, a cascade of systemic physiologic processes ensues that affect the peripheral nervous system. There is a complex interplay of local and circulating mediators, including histamine, prostaglandins, thromboxane, kinins, serotonin, catecholamines, oxygen free radicals, platelet aggregation factors, angiotensin II, and vasopressin. Initially, there is vasoconstriction at the site of injury mediated by release of norepinephrine and serotonin. A few hours after injury vasoconstriction changes to vasodilation, causing increased capillary permeability and leakage of plasma into the extravascular space. Histamine is released and damaged cells swell. Fluid shifts result in increased extravascular edema and intravascular hypovolemia. Platelets and leukocytes aggregate, leading to thrombotic ischemia.[11,12] In addition, inflammatory mediators are released. These effects lead to compromise of organ systems and, in particular, predispose the peripheral nerves to injury.

Generalized peripheral polyneuropathy is a common neurologic disorder in burn injury, with an incidence that ranges from 15% to 30%.[3,7,13] Kowalske and colleagues[5] found that age and length of intensive-care-unit stay are risk factors for developing polyneuropathies. Polyneuropathy is more commonly seen in those with greater than 20% total body surface area (TBSA) burns and electrical injuries.[14–16] Electrophysiologic evidence of polyneuropathy is commonly seen within 1 week of severe burn injury.[17] Clinically, patients may have symptoms of paresthesia and signs of mild to moderate weakness in the muscles of the distal extremities. On manual muscle testing, most patients eventually recover their strength, although they may complain of easy fatigability for years after the burn.[3,7,13] Although critical-illness neuropathy is not explicitly documented in the burn literature, severely burned patients with prolonged intensive-care-unit stays, sepsis, and multiple organ failure are at risk for critical-illness neuropathy.

Mononeuritis Multiplex

Mononeuritis multiplex is an asymmetric sensory and motor peripheral neuropathy that involves 2 or more isolated peripheral nerves. The pathophysiology is not well understood but is thought to result from a combination of circulating neurotoxins, metabolic factors, and mechanical compression. Multiple mononeuropathy was documented in 7 of 121 subjects with greater than 40% TBSA burns in 1 study.[18] In a separate study, mononeuritis multiplex was the most common diagnosis in subjects with burn injuries with a neuropathy.[14] At 1 year after injury, lower-extremity nerve lesions demonstrated better functional recovery than upper-extremity nerve lesions.[18]

Pruritus

The mechanism of pruritus is not well understood. Some investigators think it is related to axonal sprouting in the dermis and thereby classified here as a neurologic complication. Although not as devastating as some of the other neurologic manifestations of burn injuries, itch is nevertheless a significant complaint for many patients. The prevalence of pruritus is as high as 87% at 3 months and 70% at 1 year after injury.[19,20] Predictors of pruritus include deep dermal injury, extent of burn, and early posttraumatic stress symptoms.[20,21] Various treatment regimens have demonstrated a decrease in reported itch symptoms. However, a recent review examining pharmacologic and nonpharmacologic treatments of pruritus concluded that interventions lack strong empirical evidence.[22] Treatments require better clinical studies to validate their use. Nonetheless, there exist multiple clinical treatment options. Nonpharmacological treatments, including colloidal oatmeal, pulsed dye laser, silicone gels, scar massage, and transcutaneous electrical nerve stimulation, demonstrate positive effects.[22–24] Topical medications include histamine receptor antagonists and prudoxin,[25] a tricyclic antidepressant with histamine blocking properties. There are reports of the use of topical anesthetics in the treatment of pruritis.[23,26] Oral options also include selective histamine receptor antagonists and prudoxin.[27] In addition, there is preliminary evidence for use of gabapentin and ondansetron for treatment of pruritis.[28] For those with severe itching, often a combination of interventions is needed to control symptoms.

MUSCULOSKELETAL COMPLICATIONS

Musculoskeletal complications are common after burn injuries. Prevention and early identification and treatment are the goals of care in the acute, subacute, and outpatient settings. Contractures are a major musculoskeletal complication of burn injury and are covered in their own article elsewhere in this issue. The authors address bone metabolism, osteophytes, heterotopic ossification, scoliosis and kyphosis, septic arthritis, and subluxations and dislocations in detail later (**Table 3**).

Bone Metabolism

Delay in bone growth is a complication seen in the pediatric population following severe burn injury.[29] Growth disturbances result from the premature fusion of the epiphyseal plate of affected long bones. Partial epiphyseal plate fusion may also occur, causing bone deviation and deformity.[30,31] Bone-growth issues should be considered in growing children with burn scars that cross a joint and with joint contractures. In addition, case reports document that pressure garments for treatment of facial burns in children alter facial bone growth. Overbites may develop as a result of excessive pressure on the mandible. It is recommended to closely monitor facial development during and after pressure-garment use in children for development of normal dental and facial proportions.[32,33] Pressure garments may need to be modified and changed frequently to avoid these complications.

Children with burns greater than 15% TBSA exhibit decreased bone mineral density. Investigators found decreased bone mineral density at 8 weeks after injury and the loss was sustained 5 years after injury.[34] The mechanism for loss of bone mass is under investigation; however, recent research demonstrates causal roles for multiple factors, including increase in endogenous glucocorticoids, resorptive cytokines from the systemic inflammatory response, vitamin D deficiency, and disruption of calcium metabolism. Reduced bone density places children at risk for long bone fractures.[35–37] Mayes and colleagues[38] examined 104 burned children with greater than 40% TBSA and found a 5.8% incidence of fracture. Investigators have studied the use of recombinant human growth hormone without proven effect on bone formation.[39] Recent studies have demonstrated improved bone mineral density with bisphosphonate therapy. Klein and colleagues[40] performed a randomized controlled trial of 43 children with greater than 40% TBSA and examined the effects of acute administration (within 10 days of injury) of intravenous pamidronate. Subjects

Table 3
Musculoskeletal complications of burn injuries

Complication	Comments
Changes in bone metabolism	Common in children; premature fusion of epiphyseal plate of long bones; low bone mineral density in large burns
Osteophytes	Most frequent skeletal change; most common at elbow
Heterotopic ossification	Most common at elbow Risk factors: burn size, ventilator support, ICU stay, prolonged wound closure, wound infection, and graft loss
Scoliosis and kyphosis	Developed in children with asymmetric burns and contractures
Septic arthritis	Caused by penetrating burns into a joint or hematogenous seeding; associated with joint dislocation, bone and joint destruction, and restriction of movement
Subluxations and dislocations	Most common in hand and feet because of contracture formation Prevention with splinting and range of motion

receiving pamidronate demonstrated higher whole body and lumbar spine bone mineral content at discharge, 6 months, and 2 years compared with controls.[41]

Osteophytes

Evans and Smith reported that osteophytes are the most frequently observed skeletal alteration in adult patients with burn injuries. They are most often seen at the elbow and occur along the articular margins of the olecranon or coronoid process, and are thought to be caused by superimposed minor trauma to affected areas.[42,43] Pain and nerve impingement can occur depending on the size and location of the osteophytes.

Heterotopic Ossification

Heterotopic ossification is the abnormal formation of bone in soft tissue. The incidence of HO is estimated at 1% to 2% of patients who are hospitalized with burn injuries.[44–46] Clinically, only those with symptomatic joints, including impaired range of motion, joint pain, or other symptoms, require diagnostic evaluation. Therefore, reports in the literature reflect the incidence of clinically significant HO, not the true incidence. The etiology of HO is unknown. Investigators postulate that it is caused by the proliferation of primitive mesenchymal cells into osteogenic cells.[47] Other factors thought to contribute to HO include hypercalcemia, prolonged immobilization, and remobilization after prolonged immobilization.[48]

The elbow is the most frequent joint affected, comprising greater than 90% of cases in a 21-year review.[44] Risk factors associated with the development of HO include burn size, ventilator support, intensive-care-unit stay, prolonged wound closure, wound infection, and graft loss.[44,49]

HO may occur as early as 5 weeks but usually develops approximately 3 months after injury. One of the earliest signs of heterotopic ossification is loss of joint range of motion. Other clinical findings may include swelling, erythema, pain, and peripheral nerve injury. Symptoms may precede radiologic findings. A bone scan is the most sensitive diagnostic imaging test and may demonstrate positive findings up to 3 weeks before positive radiographic findings. Three-phase bone scan is limited by its low specificity; one cannot differentiate HO from other traumatic, inflammatory, or degenerative processes.[50] Plain radiographs demonstrate greater specificity than bone scan (Fig. 1).[51]

Treatment of HO begins with conservative measures, including positioning and range of motion to prevent worsening of joint motion. There are no studies examining HO prophylaxis in patients with burn injuries. However, there is evidence to support use of prophylaxis in other conditions and this data may help guide management of HO in the burn population. Nonsteroidal antiinflammatory drugs (NSAID) have proven efficacy for HO prophylaxis in patients with major hip surgery[52,53] and spinal cord injury.[54] A systematic survey of 13 randomized trials of NSAIDs used for HO prophylaxis in total hip arthroplasty showed a 57% reduction in HO in groups treated with NSAIDs.[52] Bisphosphates are effective in reducing the incidence of HO in patients with spinal cord injuries. Subjects that received oral etidronate disodium for 12 weeks after injury exhibited lower rates of HO (6%) compared with controls (27%).[55] Also, preoperative radiation of the affected hip reduces HO formation after total hip arthroplasty.[56]

Surgical intervention is reserved for treatment of symptomatic HO. Heterotopic bone that causes nerve entrapment requires timely surgical intervention to avoid permanent nerve injury. It is common practice to wait until the bone is mature before surgical intervention for HO that results in impairments in upper-extremity and lower-extremity function, mobility, and activities of daily living. HO matures over 12 to 14

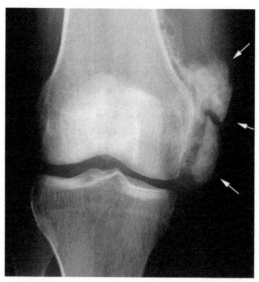

Fig. 1. Heterotopic ossification of the medial knee.

months and serial radiographs every few months are used to monitor for bone stabilization. Surgical excision of HO at the elbow results in improvement in range of motion.[57,58] Tsionos and colleagues[57] performed HO resection in 28 subjects and 35 elbows at a mean of 12 months after injury. At a mean follow-up of 21 months, flexion/extension improved from 22° preoperatively to 123° postoperatively. In a separate study of 8 children with elbow HO, all subjects demonstrated improved range of motion and were able to reach their face and perineum for functional tasks of feeding and toileting at 17 months after surgery.[58]

Scoliosis and Kyphosis

Asymmetric burns of the trunk, hips, and shoulder girdle can cause patients to favor the affected side. In the growing child, the contracture of burn scars and resultant postural change can result in structural scoliosis. In a case series, 4 children who were scalded on the back as infants developed adolescent scoliosis. The deformities of all 4 cases were corrected surgically with good results.[59] Similarly, childhood burns of the anterior neck, shoulders, and chest wall may produce a rounding of the shoulders and sunken chest. Likewise, burn-scar shortening and protective posturing can result in kyphosis. Both scoliosis and kyphosis are amenable to bracing and surgical interventions. An orthopedic surgeon is recommended to follow such patients.

Septic Arthritis

Septic arthritis is challenging to diagnose in patients who are severely burned. The characteristic signs and symptoms are often absent or masked by the overlying burn wound. Joint pain, swelling, color change, and tenderness are common symptoms at the site of burn injury or grafting and therefore are difficult to distinguish from septic arthritis.

The 2 major causes of a septic joint are penetrating burns into a joint and hematogenous seeding from bacteremia. Patients with burn injuries are at risk for infection because of their impaired immune system and concurrent illness. Septic arthritis may cause gross dislocation because of capsular laxity or cartilage and bone destruction,[60] or result in severe restriction of movement or ankylosis. It occurs most frequently in the joints of the hands, hips, knees, and wrists.

Subluxations and Dislocations

Joint subluxation of the hands and feet are common after burn injury. Burns of the dorsal surface may contract resulting in joint hyperextension. Prolonged hyperextension places the joint at risk for subluxation. This result is most common at the meta-carpophalangeal (MCP) and metatarsophalangeal (MTP) joints. Ulnar neuropathy places patients at additional risk for subluxation of the fourth and fifth digits. For dorsal hand burns, prevention of subluxation is achieved with a combination of splinting and range-of-motion exercises. A dorsal hand burn splint places the MCP joints in 60° to 90° of flexion and the distal and proximal interphalangeal joints in full extension. Similarly, the MTP joints may subluxate after contracture of healed wounds, especially in children. Application of surgical high-top shoes with a metatarsal bar helps prevent toe deformities.

Posterior hip dislocation is a problem in children. Hips maintained in an adducted and flexed position are at risk for dislocation. Anterior shoulder dislocations occur in positions of abduction and extension. Shoulder dislocations may result from positioning in the operating room.[61]

ELECTRICAL INJURIES

Electrical burn injuries are an uncommon form of burn injury, accounting for 4% of burn-unit admissions in the United States.[62] Most electrical burns result from contact with high-voltage equipment and are common at industrial worksites. The mortality rate ranges from 3% to 15%, with approximately 1000 deaths per year caused by electrical burn injuries.[62] They are the fourth leading cause of traumatic work-related deaths.[63] Similar to other burn injuries, electrical burns result in significant musculoskeletal and neurologic injuries. However, complications from electrical burn injuries differ from thermal injuries because of the particular properties of electric injuries. Types of electrical injuries and their complications are discussed later.

Etiology

There are several different types of burns that result from an electric injury. An electrical arc burn results from high-amperage currents that travel or arc through the air, typically with a high voltage difference across a gap. A massive amount of energy is released with temperatures of 2500°C to 5000°C. This release can result in a thermal burn from the high amount of energy involved, a flame burn from ignition of clothing, and a direct contact burn if the arc pathway enters the body. A flash burn occurs when the electrical arc does not enter the body; instead it causes a large surface area thermal injury. A direct contact burn occurs when the person becomes part of the circuit, with electricity passing from the contact point through their body to an exit point. The electricity causes electrothermal burns at the entry and exit point, and also through the deep tissue involved in its path (**Fig. 2**). This type of injury is particularly devastating because the path often involves vital tissues, nerves, and organs.

Electrical burn injuries are categorized by voltage; greater than 1000 V is classified as a high-voltage or high-tension injury and less than 1000 V is classified as a low-voltage or low-tension injury. Low-tension injuries are common in the home or office setting. A classic case is the child that bites an electrical cord resulting in oral burns. The severity of an electrical burn is related to the amount of current. Ohm's Law states that current is directly proportional to voltage and indirectly proportional to resistance.

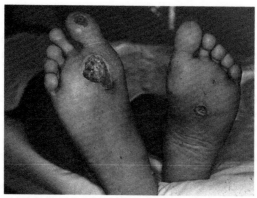

Fig. 2. Electrical injury with entry and exit points of the feet.

Therefore, a high-tension injury through an area of the body with the lowest resistance will cause the maximum amount of tissue damage.

Neurologic Complications

Low-tension and high-tension injuries result in different neurologic complications. Low-tension alternating current, the standard mode of electrical delivery in the world, causes muscle tetany that can increase contact time with the electrical source. In contrast, high-tension circuits are often completed by arcing. High voltage results in a massive contraction of muscles that can throw the victim and reduce contact time. In some cases low-tension alternating current injuries cause more neurologic injury than high-tension injuries because of longer contact time. However, in the majority of cases severe neurologic consequences of electrical burns are caused by high-tension injuries as a result of their high-energy involvement. Neurologic complications occur in up to 70% of electrical injuries.[16]

Neuropsychological Sequelae

Loss of consciousness is the most common neurologic sequela of electrical injury, occurring in 40% of the population.[16,64] Most cases experience a transient loss of consciousness and this is associated with a favorable prognosis. In contrast, a greater than 10 minute loss of consciousness is associated with intracranial damage and exhibits a worse prognosis.[64] Independent of loss of consciousness, survivors report other neuropsychological problems immediately following injury, including severe headaches, ataxia, blindness, deafness, aphasia, and delirium. These findings are usually transient and without long-term affects.[64] In a recent study of 39 subjects with electrical injuries, Singerman[65] found numbness, weakness, memory problems, paresthesias, and chronic pain were the most prevalent long-term neurologic sequelae. A total of 71% of subjects also experienced psychological complications. The most common psychological symptoms were anxiety, nightmares, and insomnia.[65] Other investigators documented long-term psychological consequences, including depression, sexual dysfunction, reduced attention, posttraumatic stress disorder, and lack of motivation after electric injury.[66]

Peripheral Neuropathy

Peripheral neuropathy can result from both high-tension and low-tension injuries, with prevalence as high as 30%.[67] Nerve damage can occur by direct contact with electrical current or entrapment caused by postinjury changes. Contact burns located near nerves can damage the axons or the neurovascular bundle by thermal injury. Return of neurologic function is expected with sparing of the nerve sheath and vasculature. Neuropathies may also occur as a result of tissue edema and coagulation necrosis that leads to nerve entrapment.[68] Severe compression of blood vessels by compartment syndrome causes ischemic necrosis of the tissues, including nerves. In this situation, all nerves in the affected area are involved.[69] Peripheral neuropathy is also associated with scar-tissue development around or within the peripheral nerve, either obstructing regeneration of a damaged nerve or causing a new compression neuropathy.[68] Similar to traditional burn injuries, swelling of burned tissue can cause entrapment of nerves at specific anatomic sites that are predisposed to compression. Specifically, the median nerve can be entrapped at the carpal tunnel, the ulnar nerve at Guyon's canal or the cubital tunnel, and the posterior interosseous nerve at the Arcade of Frohse.[70] Contact burns to the palmar surface may result in median and ulnar nerve injuries.[68]

Low-tension injuries cause peripheral neuropathy with prolonged contact caused by tetany or with lowered skin resistance caused by water. Such nerve injuries are associated with the location of the current, not necessarily the location of the burn. Brachial plexopathies are documented with current passing from hand to hand.[68,71] Investigators postulate that perineural fibrosis plays a pathophysiologic role in low-tension peripheral nerve injuries.[72]

Spinal Cord Injuries

Spinal cord injuries are an uncommon but significant complication of electrical burn injury, with an incidence of 2% to 5%.[73] These injuries result from fall or blunt force trauma related to the electrical injury, or as a result of electrical current. There are case reports of direct electrical injury to the spinal cord with high-tension injuries resulting in paraparesis and quadriparesis with motor and sensory involvement.[16] Also, there are reports of delayed onset spinal cord injuries associated with electrical injuries. In such cases, symptoms develop from 2 days to 2 years after the initial injury.[74] Delayed spinal cord injuries exhibit poor prognosis for neurologic recovery. In a review of 40 subjects with delayed spinal cord injury, 2 subjects demonstrated partial recovery.[75] Pathophysiology of delayed spinal cord injuries is poorly understood but it is postulated that there is thermal and vascular damage to the spinal cord from the electrical injury.[73]

Musculoskeletal Complications

Electrical burn injuries impact the musculoskeletal system. In the acute phase fractures, compartment syndrome and amputations are common. In one case series of 50 subjects with electrical injuries over a 7-year period, 40% demonstrated musculoskeletal injuries with 11% requiring multiple amputations.[67] Musculoskeletal complications often require rehabilitative care and affect survivors' functional outcomes.

Fractures

Fractures occur as a direct result of trauma from electrical injuries. High-tension injuries can throw the victim from the source of electricity, causing trauma by fall or blunt force. Falls are often related to the location of the electrical source and occur from transformer towers, electrical poles, and rooftops.[76] Muscle contraction and tetany induced by electrical injuries can generate enough force to dislocate or fracture bones.[77]

Muscle Ischemia and Amputation

Deep muscle injury and necrosis occur as a result of high-tension injuries. Bone exhibits a high resistance compared with other tissues, and therefore a high amount of heat is dissipated in bony areas.[78] Given its proximity to electric current, muscle is predisposed to severe thermal injury with ensuing muscle necrosis. Muscle necrosis can lead to edema, elevation in intracompartment pressure, and subsequent compartment syndrome. The route of electrical current often spares the skin that is superficial to the area of muscle necrosis and can lead to unrecognized deep tissue injury. Some authors advocate routine exploration of deep muscle compartments for high-tension injuries.[79] Early escharotomy and fasciotomy may prevent subsequent amputation as a result of compartment syndrome.[80] Significant muscle and tissue necrosis at distal extremities, usually the sites of entry and exit of the electrical current, may require amputation.[81,82] Rai[81] reviewed 58 high-tension electrical burns and found that amputation and deep muscle injuries were the most common complications. A total of 33% of subjects required amputation and an additional 29% experienced deep muscle injuries that did not require amputation. Amputations are less common with low-tension injuries. Hussman[83] reviewed 91 subjects with low-tension injuries and found an amputation rate of 1%. All amputations involved digits and there were no major limb amputations. Significant muscle necrosis also leads to rhabdomyolysis, a common renal complication of electrical injuries.

Other Bony Changes

Electrical injuries cause periosteal new bone formation, bone splitting, and bony necrosis.[82] After amputation, new bone formation is seen at residual limb long bones. Helm and Walker[84] reviewed 61 amputation sites in 43 burn survivors with electrical injuries. A total of 23 of 28 subjects with long-bone amputations developed new bone formation at the amputation site. No new bone growth was evidenced in the 15 subjects with small-bone amputations and disarticulations. The average time from amputation to diagnosis of new bone formation was 38 weeks. Of those with new bone formation, 12% required surgical revision of the residual limb, and 7% required replacement of their prosthesis secondary to new bone formation. The etiology of new bone formation in the electrical amputee is unknown.

Bone splitting, swelling, and necrosis are related to electrical current passes through bone. Vrabec and Kolar[82] described these changes occurring from inflammatory reactions caused by avulsion of the periosteum from electrical injury.

SUMMARY

As more people survive burn injuries, there is an increasing focus on managing the complications of burn injuries with the ultimate goal of improving survivors' quality of life. Musculoskeletal and neurologic sequelae are significant complications of burn injury. Electrical injury is a subcategory of burns with multiple musculoskeletal and neurologic complications. Knowledge of these complications helps clinicians provide optimal long-term care for burn survivors and enables survivors to attain maximal recovery.

REFERENCES

1. American Burn Association. Burn incidence and treatment in the US: 2007 fact sheet. Available at: www.ameriburn.org/resources_factsheet.php. Accessed September 1, 2010.

2. Ryan CM, Schoenfeld DA, Thorpe WP, et al. Objective estimates of the probability of death from burn injuries. N Engl J Med 1998;338(6):362–6.
3. Henderson B, Koepke GH, Feller I. Peripheral polyneuropathy among patients with burns. Arch Phys Med Rehabil 1971;52(4):149–51.
4. Helm PA, Ralph Johnson E, McIntosh Carlton A. Peripheral neurological problems in the acute burn patient. Burns 1977;3(2):123–5.
5. Kowalske K, Holavanahalli R, Helm P. Neuropathy after burn injury. J Burn Care Rehabil 2001;22:353–7.
6. Helm PA, Pandian G, Heck E. Neuromuscular problems in the burn patient: cause and prevention. Arch Phys Med Rehabil 1985;66(7):451–3.
7. Jackson L, Keats AS. Mechanism of brachial plexus palsy following anesthesia. Anesthesiology 1965;26:190–4.
8. Aho K, Sainio K, Kianta M, et al. Pneumatic tourniquet paralysis. Case report. J Bone Joint Surg Br 1983;65(4):441–3.
9. Reinstein L, Alevizatos AC, Twardzik FG, et al. Femoral nerve dysfunction after retroperitoneal hemorrhage: pathophysiology revealed by computed tomography. Arch Phys Med Rehabil 1984;65(1):37–40.
10. Lee MY, Liu G, Kowlowitz V, et al. Causative factors affecting peripheral neuropathy in burn patients. Burns 2009;35(3):412–6.
11. Kramer GC, Nguyen T. Pathophysiology of burn shock and burn edema. In: Herndon DN, editor. Total burn care. London: W.B. Saunders; 1997. p. 44–52.
12. Johnson C. Pathologic manifestations of burn injury. In: Richard R, Staley MA, editors. Burn care and rehabilitation: principles and practice. Philadelphia: F.A. Davis; 1994. p. 29–48.
13. Helm P. Neuromuscular considerations. In: Fisher SV, Helm P, editors. Comprehensive rehabilitation of burns. Baltimore (MD): Williams and Wilkins; 1984. p. 235–41.
14. Khedr EM, Khedr T, el-Oteify MA, et al. Peripheral neuropathy in burn patients. Burns 1997;23(7/8):579–83.
15. Marquez S, Turley JJ, Peters WJ. Neuropathy in burn patients. Brain 1993; 116(Pt 2):471–83.
16. Grube BJ, Heimbach DM, Engrav LH, et al. Neurologic consequences of electrical burns. J Trauma Inj Infect Crit Care 1990;30(3):254–8.
17. Margherita AJ, Robinson LR, Heimbach DM, et al. Burn-associated peripheral polyneuropathy. A search for causative factors. Am J Phys Med Rehabil 1995; 74(1):28–32.
18. Dagum AB, Peters WJ, Neligan PC, et al. Severe multiple mononeuropathy in patients with major thermal burns. J Burn Care Rehabil 1993;14(4):440–5.
19. Willebrand M, Low A, Dyster-Aas J, et al. Pruritus, personality traits and coping in long-term follow-up of burn-injured patients. Acta Derm Venereol 2004;84(5): 375–80.
20. Van Loey NE, Bremer M, Faber AW, et al. Itching following burns: epidemiology and predictors. Br J Dermatol 2008;158(1):95–100.
21. Vitale M, Fields-Blache C, Luterman A. Severe itching in the patient with burns. J Burn Care Rehabil 1991;12(4):330–3.
22. Bell PL, Gabriel V. Evidence based review for the treatment of post-burn pruritus [review]. J Burn Care Res 2009;30(1):55–61.
23. Matheson JD, Clayton J, Muller MJ. The reduction of itch during burn wound healing. J Burn Care Rehabil 2001;22(1):76–81.
24. Hettrick HH, O'Brien K, Laznick H, et al. Effect of transcutaneous electrical nerve stimulation for the management of burn pruritus: a pilot study. J Burn Care Rehabil 2004;25(3):236–40.

25. Eschler DC, Klein PA. An evidence-based review of the efficacy of topical antihistamines in the relief of pruritus [review]. J Drugs Dermatol 2010;9(8):992–7.
26. Kopecky EA, Jacobson S, Bch MB, et al. Safety and pharmacokinetics of EMLA in the treatment of postburn pruritus in pediatric patients: a pilot study. J Burn Care Rehabil 2001;22(3):235–42.
27. Pour-Reza-Gholi F, Nasrollahi A, Firouzan A, et al. Low-dose doxepin for treatment of pruritus in patients on hemodialysis. Iran J Kidney Dis 2007;1(1):34–7.
28. Goutos I, Dziewulski P, Richardson PM. Pruritus in burns: review article [review]. J Burn Care Res 2009;30:221–8.
29. Prelack K, Dwyer J, Dallal GE, et al. Growth deceleration and restoration after serious burn injury. J Burn Care Res 2007;28(2):262–8.
30. Jackson D MacG. Destructive burns: some orthopaedic complications. Burns 1980;7(2):105–22.
31. Reed MH. Growth disturbances in the hands following thermal injuries in children. 2. Frostbite [review]. Can Assoc Radiol J 1988;39(2):95–9.
32. Leung KS, Cheng JC, Ma GF, et al. Complications of pressure therapy for postburn hypertrophic scars. Biomechanical analysis based on 5 patients. Burns Incl Therm Inj 1984;10(6):434–8.
33. Fricke NB, Omnell ML, Dutcher KA, et al. Skeletal and dental disturbances in children after facial burns and pressure garment use: a 4-year follow-up. J Burn Care Rehabil 1999;20(3):239–49.
34. Klein GL, Herndon DN, Langman CB, et al. Long-term reduction in bone mass after severe burn injury in children. J Pediatr 1995;126(2):252–6.
35. Klein GL, Bi LX, Sherrard DJ, et al. Evidence supporting a role of glucocorticoids in short-term bone loss in burned children. Osteoporos Int 2004;15(6):468–74.
36. Klein GL, Langman CB, Herndon DN. Vitamin D depletion following burn injury in children: a possible factor in post-burn osteopenia. J Trauma Inj Infect Crit Care 2002;52(2):346–50.
37. Klein GL, Herndon DN, Goodman WG, et al. Histomorphometric and biochemical characterization of bone following acute severe burns in children. Bone 1995; 17(5):455–60.
38. Mayes T, Gottschlich M, Scanlon J, et al. Four-year review of burns as an etiologic factor in the development of long bone fractures in pediatric patients. J Burn Care Rehabil 2003;24(5):279–84.
39. Klein GL, Wolf SE, Langman CB, et al. Effects of therapy with recombinant human growth hormone on insulin-like growth factor system components and serum levels of biochemical markers of bone formation in children after severe burn injury. J Clin Endocrinol Metab 1998;83(1):21–4.
40. Klein GL, Wimalawansa SJ, Kulkarni G, et al. The efficacy of acute administration of pamidronate on the conservation of bone mass following severe burn injury in children: a double-blind, randomized, controlled study. Osteoporos Int 2005; 16(6):631–5.
41. Przkora R, Herndon DN, Sherrard DJ, et al. Pamidronate preserves bone mass for at least 2 years following acute administration for pediatric burn injury. Bone 2007;41(2):297–302.
42. Evans EB, Smith JR. Bone and joint changes following burns; a roentgenographic study; preliminary report. J Bone Joint Surg Am 1959;41(5):785–99.
43. Evans E. Bone and joint changes secondary to burns. In: Lynch JB, Lewis SR, editors. Symposium on the treatment of burns. St Louis (MO): CV Mosby; 1973. p. 76–8.
44. Hunt JL, Arnoldo BD, Kowalske K, et al. Heterotopic ossification revisited: a 21-year surgical experience. J Burn Care Res 2006;27(4):535–40.

45. Peterson SL, Mani MM, Crawford CM, et al. Postburn heterotopic ossification: insights for management decision making. J Trauma Inj Infect Crit Care 1989; 29(3):365–9.

46. Elledge ES, Smith AA, McManus WF, et al. Heterotopic bone formation in burned patients. J Trauma Inj Infect Crit Care 1988;28(5):684–7.

47. Urist MR, Nakagawa M, Nakata N, et al. Experimental myositis ossificans: cartilage and bone formation in muscle in response to a diffusible bone matrix-derived morphogen. Arch Pathol Lab Med 1978;102(6):312–6.

48. Shehab D, Elgazzar AH, Collier BD. Heterotopic ossification [review]. J Nucl Med 2002;43(3):346–53.

49. Klein MB, Logsetty S, Costa B, et al. Extended time to wound closure is associated with increased risk of heterotopic ossification of the elbow. J Burn Care Res 2007;28(3):447–50.

50. van Kuijk AA, Geurts AC, van Kuppevelt HJ. Neurogenic heterotopic ossification in spinal cord injury [review]. Spinal Cord 2002;40(7):313–26.

51. Freed JH, Hahn H, Menter R, et al. The use of the three-phase bone scan in the early diagnosis of heterotopic ossification and in the evaluation of Didronel therapy. Paraplegia 1982;20:208–16.

52. Neal BC, Rodgers A, Clark T, et al. A systematic survey of 13 randomized trials of non-steroidal anti-inflammatory drugs for the prevention of heterotopic bone formation after major hip surgery [review]. Acta Orthop Scand 2000;71(2):122–8.

53. Schmidt SA, Kjaersgaard-Andersen P, Pedersen NW, et al. The use of indomethacin to prevent the formation of heterotopic bone after total hip replacement. A randomized, double-blind clinical trial. J Bone Joint Surg Am 1988;70(6):834–8.

54. Banovac K, Williams JM, Patrick LD, et al. Prevention of heterotopic ossification after spinal cord injury with COX-2 selective inhibitor (rofecoxib). Spinal Cord 2004;42(12):707–10.

55. Finerman GA, Stover SL. Heterotopic ossification following hip replacement or spinal cord injury. Two clinical studies with EHDP. Metab Bone Dis Relat Res 1981;3(4/5):337–42.

56. Pellegrini VD Jr, Gregoritch SJ. Preoperative irradiation for prevention of heterotopic ossification following total hip arthroplasty. J Bone Joint Surg Am 1996; 78(6):870–81.

57. Tsionos I, Leclercq C, Rochet JM. Heterotopic ossification of the elbow in patients with burns. Results after early excision. J Bone Joint Surg Br 2004; 86(3):396–403.

58. Gaur A, Sinclair M, Caruso E, et al. Heterotopic ossification around the elbow following burns in children: results after excision. J Bone Joint Surg Am 2003; 85(8):1538–43.

59. Qiu Y, Wang SF, Wang B, et al. Adolescent scar contracture scoliosis caused by back scalding during the infantile period. Eur Spine J 2007;16(10):1557–62.

60. Kim A, Palmieri TL, Greenhalgh DG, et al. Septic hip presenting with dislocation as a source of occult infection in a burn patient. J Burn Care Res 2006;27(5): 749–52.

61. Hinton AE, King D. Anterior shoulder dislocation as a complication of surgery for burns. Burns 1989;15(4):248–9.

62. Lee RC. Injury by electrical forces: pathophysiology, manifestations, and therapy [review]. Curr Probl Surg 1997;34(9):677–764.

63. Casini V. Worker deaths by electrocution: a summary of NIOSH surveillance and investigative findings. Cincinnati (OH): National Institute for Occupational Safety and Health; 1998. p. 5–8.

64. Leibovici D, Shemer J, Shapira SC. Electrical injuries: current concepts. Injury 1995;26(9):623–7.
65. Singerman J, Gomez M, Fish JS. Long-term sequelae of low-voltage electrical injury. J Burn Care Res 2008;29(5):773–7.
66. Morse JS, Morse MS. Diffuse electrical injury: comparison of physical and neuro-psychological symptom presentation in males and females. J Psychosom Res 2005;58(1):51–4.
67. Ferreiro I, Meléndez J, Regalado J, et al. Factors influencing the sequelae of high tension electrical injuries. Burns 1998;24(7):649–53.
68. Fish RM. Electric injury, Part II: specific injuries. J Emerg Med 2000;18(1):27–34.
69. Rempel D, Dahlin L, Lundborg G. Pathophysiology of nerve compression syndromes: response of peripheral nerves to loading [review]. J Bone Joint Surg Am 1999;81(11):1600–10.
70. Winkelman MD. Neurological complications of thermal and electrical burns. In: Aminoff MJ, editor. Neurology and general medicine. 4th edition. Philadelphia: Churchill Livingstone; 2008. p. 1031–43.
71. Suematsu N, Matsuura J, Atsuta Y. Brachial plexus injury caused by electric current through the ulnar nerve. Case report and review of the literature [review]. Arch Orthop Trauma Surg 1989;108(6):400–2.
72. Smith MA, Muehlberger T, Dellon AL. Peripheral nerve compression associated with low-voltage electrical injury without associated significant cutaneous burn. Plast Reconstr Surg 2002;109(1):137–44.
73. Varghese G, Mani MM, Redford JB. Spinal cord injuries following electrical accidents. Paraplegia 1986;24(3):159–66.
74. Christensen JA, Sherman RT, Balis GA, et al. Delayed neurologic injury secondary to high-voltage current, with recovery. J Trauma Inj Infect Crit Care 1980;20(2):166–8.
75. Levine NS, Atkins A, McKeel DW Jr, et al. Spinal cord injury following electrical accidents: case reports. J Trauma Inj Infect Crit Care 1975;15(5):459–63.
76. Maghsoudi H, Adyani Y, Ahmadian N. Electrical and lightning injuries. J Burn Care Res 2007;28(2):255–61.
77. Koumbourlis AC. Electrical injuries [review]. Crit Care Med 2002;30(Suppl 11): S424–30.
78. Chilbert M, Maiman D, Sances A Jr, et al. Measure of tissue resistivity in experi-mental electrical burns. J Trauma Inj Infect Crit Care 1985;25(3):209–15.
79. d'Amato TA, Kaplan IB, Britt LD. High-voltage electrical injury: a role for manda-tory exploration of deep muscle compartments. J Natl Med Assoc 1994;86(7): 535–7.
80. Kopp J, Loos B, Spilker G, et al. Correlation between serum creatinine kinase levels and extent of muscle damage in electrical burns. Burns 2004;30(7):680–3.
81. Rai J, Jeschke MG, Barrow RE, et al. Electrical injuries: a 30-year review. J Trauma Inj Infect Crit Care 1999;46(5):933–6.
82. Vrabec R, Kolar J. Bone changes caused by electrical current. In: Transactions of the fourth international congress of plastic and reconstructive surgery. Rome (Italy): Excerpta Medica; 1969. p. 215–7.
83. Hussmann J, Kucan JO, Russell RC, et al. Electrical injuries–morbidity, outcome and treatment rationale. Burns 1995;21:530–5.
84. Helm PA, Walker SC. New bone formation at amputation sites in electrically burn-injured patients. Arch Phys Med Rehabil 1987;68(5 Pt 1):284–6.

Prosthetic Management of the Burn Amputation

John R. Fergason, BA, CPO*, Ryan Blanck, BS, CPO

KEYWORDS

- Amputation • Microprocessor • Transradial
- Transhumeral • Shear

Many amputations are sustained as a result of trauma and the associated complications. When burns are the cause of amputation, the difficulty of the rehabilitation significantly increases. Often the burn-related amputation will maintain the presence of tissue and bone characteristics that complicate the fitting of a prosthetic device. These characteristics often include grafted skin, creative muscle flaps to attain surface coverage, skin adhesions, and continuous tissue breakdown. Because of the difficulty of these cases, this specific population may experience the most measurable benefit from a multidisciplinary approach to upper and lower extremity amputee rehabilitation. The most successful rehabilitation outcome will occur when the team has a collective understanding of burn tissue dynamics and healing progression and access to the available prosthetic technology. Most patients with burn amputations can still experience successful prosthetic use, particularly if they have only single amputations of the lower limb.[1,2] Team members should be able to draw from past experiences and realize that each patient may require unique new or varying prosthetic design adaptations. Communication from each team member will play a crucial role in the progression of the patient's overall functional abilities.

In addition, burn-related amputations are often combined with other associated injuries that contribute to the complicated polytrauma nature of the care. Also important to remember is that most cases seen by the Department of Defense will eventually require care and services from the Department of Veterans Affairs or private sector. Amputees with compromised burn tissue may not always have easy access to this care. Even today, access to appropriate prosthetic care and associated ongoing or necessary rehabilitation services may be challenging in some areas of the country. Given this scenario, patients should be taught to self-advocate for their care and be educated on socket design, interfaces, componentry, and associated technology. Having this knowledge will help them to successfully identify and communicate issues to their future care providers.

The authors have nothing to disclose.
Department of Orthopedics and Rehabilitation, Brooke Army Medical Center, Center for the Intrepid, 3851 Roger Brooke Drive, Fort Sam Houston, TX 78234, USA
* Corresponding author.
E-mail address: john.fergason@amedd.army.mil

Phys Med Rehabil Clin N Am 22 (2011) 277–299
doi:10.1016/j.pmr.2011.03.001
1047-9651/11/$ – see front matter. Published by Elsevier Inc.

PRE-PROSTHETIC EVALUATION AND TRAINING
Electrical Versus Thermal Mechanisms

Severe thermal and electrical burns can result in amputations with similar characteristics, even though the mechanism of injury is different. Electrical and thermal burn injuries may present with several key differences (**Fig. 1**). Electrical burns from high-voltage contact are associated with longer hospital stays and more complex surgical procedures.[3] Electrical injuries treated with an early faciotomy have an increased incidence of developing deep venous thrombosis and requiring an amputation.[4] These injuries also have an increased prevalence of deep tissue destruction, nerve damage, severe ischemia, and delayed hemorrhage that may compromise future fittings, particularly in the upper extremity.[5,6]

If a myoelectric system is desired, nerve compromise not only can cause strength and range of motion issues but also may present with reduced efficiency of the electromyogram signals needed for myoelectric control systems. Furthermore, cognitive/brain issues related to entry or exit of the high voltage electrical injury may be possible. Many cases have bilateral upper extremity involvement from the natural tendency for dual-hand grasping of live electrical wires by individuals working around high voltage. Entry and exit areas of high-voltage electrocution injuries have an increased potential for lower extremity damage. One retrospective study showed that free-flap coverage performed as a secondary procedure in flame, contact, or fluid burns had a higher success rate, suggesting that timing of the procedure was correlated to the successful outcome.[7] In terms of the decision to amputate, early identification of nonsalvageable limbs has been shown to decrease infections and improve the mortality rate.[8]

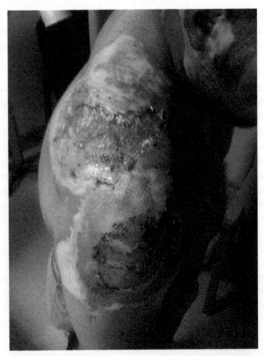

Fig. 1. Transradial amputation at the exit site resulting from an electrocution injury.

Range of Motion Limitations

Range-of-motion limitations often occur because the surface and underlying soft tissues are adherent and lose elasticity; this is especially true in the presence of skin grafts. Range-of-motion deficits are particularly limiting in the upper and lower extremities when they are short of functional range. To reduce their functional effect on performance, some limitations can be compensated for through alignment and with particular prosthetic components. Adherent skin can be limiting in the lower extremity because the protections afforded by skin elasticity are not present in weight-bearing conditions. In the upper extremity, protection over the bony prominences is compromised, as is sensation, which is helpful in proprioceptive feedback. One large prospective study found that 38.7% of 985 burn patients developed at least one contracture at hospital discharge. Amputation was one of the primary predictors of the severity of a contracture.[9]

Sensation Compromise

As expected, sensation is rarely normal in most burn patients. Grafted skin is considerably thinner than normal skin and has reduced underlying soft tissue. This thinned and compromised soft tissue envelope has an increased potential for hypersensitivity. This skin needs adequate time to heal, but some patients may become apprehensive about touching the limb because of hypersensitivity. Burn patients can also develop hyposensitivity and hypersensitivity. Hypersensitivity can limit the ability to comfortably don and doff the prosthesis and use compression dressings or the liners often incorporated into the prosthetic design. Some patients who present with hypersensitivity of the limb may also have zones of decreased sensation or hyposensitivity. This occurrence can become a problem for patients who are familiar with issues surrounding a hypersensitive part of the limb but are unaware of an area of hyposensitivity, because this can lead to the unknowing development of a skin breakdown secondary to contributors, such as sleeping pressures or compression garments. This hyposensitivity can eventually result in lack of protection from the dangers of friction and pressure within the prosthesis.

The level of sensation present and how it can be interpreted can be determined with simple monofilament sensation mapping. Although the Semmes-Weinstein monofilaments are designed for the plantar surface of the foot, they can be helpful in establishing relative levels of sensation (**Fig. 2**), which can be particularly helpful when eliciting feedback on the comfort of the prosthesis. If the clinician and patient know where the sensation is reliable, the feedback will be much more consistent and valuable. When patients can tangibly see how limited their sensation is, they are more inclined to take precautions to prevent fitting problems in the limb that can lead to skin breakdown.

PATIENT GOALS
Desensitization

Early association of the patient with the amputation is an important step in the desensitization process. Many patients develop an early tendency to avoid contact and even viewing their amputations, which may increase the potential for hypersensitivity and create challenges to comfortable interfacing with the initial prosthetic system. Burn patients may also have an increased potential for limb avoidance because of the nature of the injury and valid levels of pain associated with the extended healing process. Progressive use of ace wraps, residual limb shrinkers, or gel roll-on liners can aid in the desensitization process and help patients interact with their new

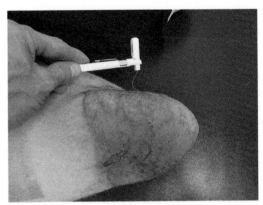

Fig. 2. Semmes-Weinstein monofilaments can be used to determine relative levels of sensation on the weight-bearing regions of the residual limb.

amputation early and directly. The independent donning and doffing of shrinkers and liners can be great initial exposure to the future world of daily prosthetic use.

Simple limb manipulation and massage should also be implemented early. The discomfort associated with the early limb desensitization process can be eased through performing manipulation over and through the compression garment or liner. This process also prevents interference with the various wound care techniques, such as medications and dressings, that are being implemented on the skin. Occasionally, custom-designed silicon interfacing has been required even at the preprosthetic early stage of treatment because of the shape, range of motion, and state of skin integrity of the burned residual limb. The custom interfaces can be molded, fabricated, and fit on site to expedite the process and maintain the treatment progression for the patient (**Fig. 3**).

Education and Goal Setting

Even in the very early healing phase of rehabilitation, many patients express their desire for the most advanced prosthetic system possible. It is important for clinicians to help them understand that the initial prosthesis may either have advanced technology or be a more simple design, and often is some combination of both. The patient must trust the prosthetist and the treating team to understand the reasoning behind the component choices. Building early rapport with the patient and family gives them the confidence that the treatment team can be trusted to keep the patient's best interest at the center of the prescription development for the first limb. The prosthetic options seem limitless and confusing at first, and may be complicated by misinformation obtained from Web searches, personal anecdotes, and well-meaning testimonials. However, the prosthetist and treating team members must also be empathetic and listen to the opinions, desires, and goals of the patient from day one.

Family and Peer Influences

During this early phase of treatment, it is beneficial for the patient and family to begin understanding various aspects of the fit and function of the initial prosthetic system that may be used. Several sessions may be recommended to gradually introduce the patient to current technology options and the concepts behind the progression of prosthetic care within the first 9 to 12 months of treatment. With burn amputees, the family, involved friends, and caregivers must be encouraged to actively participate

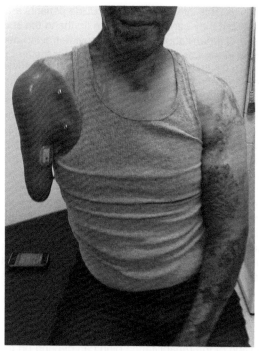

Fig. 3. Custom silicone liners can be fabricated by the prosthetist to accommodate shape anomalies and increase skin protection. Liner for a myoelectrically controlled transhumeral prosthesis is shown.

in the early prosthetic education to help clarify their role in the rehabilitation process. By this time, many family and friends have supported these patients with 24-hour care, and this commitment is a significant one. Family members can be educated on all aspects of the patient's rehabilitation, including simple things from use of dressings under shrinkers and liners, donning of the prostheses, skin checks, and function of a myoelectric prosthesis, among a variety of other related aspects of prosthetic use and rehabilitation.

A difficult new and unexpected challenge becomes apparent when the patient discharges to an outpatient setting. Without professional 24-hour acute care, patients and family must learn how to gradually rely less on others and increase personal independence. Because each patient will react differently, an understanding of that patient's cultural view of disability, severity of injury, location of family, and even the circumstance of the injury must be well understood. Family dynamics are different for each case, therefore a family meeting to discuss the rehabilitation goals and plan of progression for use and eventual independence can be very helpful for all parties involved.

Unlike amputations that are secondary to disease processes, traumatic amputations are unplanned, and leave patients little or no time to process the situation. Amputations that are burn-related are often performed in emergent circumstances, and these patients are suddenly introduced, through no choice of their own, to the world of amputation and prosthetic devices. They often feel very isolated and like no one could possibly understand their circumstances. One helpful approach is to introduce these patients to someone who has at least a similar amputation level and has completed rehabilitation. This introduction can provide patients an opportunity to talk with someone with whom they can relate and see firsthand the successful outcomes of rehabilitation. Several organizations can help provide trained peer counselors who are prepared to assist in the transition to or preparing for the first prosthesis.

Medical Justification

In addition to the normal preprosthetic goals and education, preparation for medical justification can begin as early as the day of injury. Education on medical justification includes all treatment providers involved with care of the patient. Experiences and findings of each team member can provide valuable information when formulating a thorough and appropriate medical justification, not only for the initial prosthesis but also those that will follow soon after. Many insurance carriers require that a typical upper-extremity amputee first use standard conventional systems before a myoelectric or hybrid system. The main reasons for this are related to cost and the understanding that in the past many upper-extremity amputees discontinue use of their first prosthesis. Burn amputees may require more advanced upper extremity myoelectric technology earlier than some insurance carriers are accustomed to considering. The more clinical information coupled with published evidence that can be provided to the insurance carrier, the more likely the recommended and prescribed prosthesis will be covered.

PROSTHETIC PRESCRIPTION: APPROACH AND PROGRESSION

Successful progression of the rehabilitation plan can depend on the appropriateness of the first prosthetic prescription. Prescriptions that are developed systematically to address specific patient characteristics will provide patients the best opportunity to progress with the rehabilitation team. Skin issues are the most common characteristic that need special attention. All prosthetic devices will have some amount of movement, because the prosthesis is used in a functional range of motion. This movement will have both shear and slip associated with it, and may at some point cause skin breakdown. Careful distribution of socket pressure in load-tolerant areas will help maintain skin integrity. Sustained forces through an area with minimal soft tissue coverage or adhesion of tissue to underlying bony anatomy can incur skin breakdown fairly rapidly. Given the compromise in protective sensation for most patients, they can be unaware of the presence of pressure or shear that can lead to breakdown.

In all prosthetic fittings, a well-planned progressive wearing schedule is vital to minimizing complications with skin and load/force-tolerance issues. The wearing schedule protocol requirements must be followed even more stringently than in the population with uncompromised skin. The patient, family, and caregivers must understand that even with the a well-designed and properly fitting prosthesis, early fittings over burned and grafted residual limb tissue will normally have incidence of breakdown and complications. This breakdown can be caused even just from the donning and doffing of the limb. Using lubricants on areas where shear is expected is a simple method to reduce this risk (**Fig. 4**). These incidences of breakdown can be considered normal and expected as the skin heals, matures, and changes in its structure and quality.

The early fitting process can be delayed too long when waiting for ideal skin before proceeding with fitting of the initial prosthesis. Studies have retrospectively shown that the duration of preprosthetic fitting time can significantly affect the satisfaction and daily use time of the prosthesis.[10] Therefore, efforts should be made to accelerate the process when possible (**Fig. 5**). This concept can be difficult for many on the treatment team to understand and be comfortable with, although this does not mean that

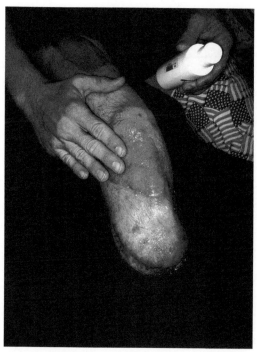

Fig. 4. Hypoallergenic lubricants are used to reduce shear over compromised regions of the limb before donning the prosthesis.

a skin issue that is getting larger, deeper, or showing signs of infection should be tolerated or ignored by the patient or treatment team. In the authors' experience, educating the patient, therapists, and physicians on why a particular skin complication has developed and how it can be controlled, enables therapy to be cautiously resumed under strict supervision by all providers. However, occasions will still arise that require patients to limit or completely stop the use of a prosthesis because of more significant skin complications, postoperative healing issues, or even pending surgical procedures. At this point the patient should be informed about the reasoning for stoppage and the potential timeline that may be expected before prosthetic adjustment or refitting can occur. Again this shows how critical it is to have a well-developed professional relationship between all caregivers involved.

PROSTHETIC PRESCRIPTION FOR THE LOWER EXTREMITY
Socket

The socket is the primary supporting aspect of the prosthesis, thus the design deserves particular attention with the burn patient. Monofilament testing can be used to determine what weight-bearing regions of the residual limb have protective sensation and can be safely used. For example, if a patella tendon–bearing design is desired for a transtibial amputation, the weight-bearing regions include the patella tendon, medial tibial flare, pretibial region, gastrocsoleus, and popliteal space.[11] Muscle flaps and skin grafting have been shown to be effective in providing soft tissue coverage of the below-knee burn amputation, but the ability to use these more common weight-bearing area of the limb may be compromised.[12,13] Several concepts

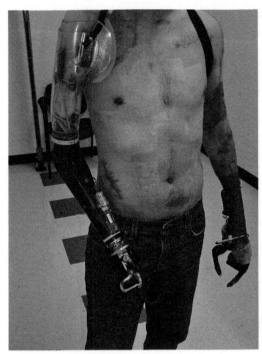

Fig. 5. Early prosthetic fitting enabled independence on this bilateral patient with transhumeral and partial hand amputations.

taken into account include the force coupling nature of the pressure when ambulating, the vertical components of weight support, and the ability of the skin to tolerate shear.

If a particular region of the limb is weighted, a counterforce in the opposite region of the limb will also be necessary. Both regions must be capable of appropriate tolerance to pressure. An alternative to the patella tendon–bearing design is the use of a total surface-bearing socket. This design uses weight-bearing in a more hydrostatic manner to reduce weight-bearing focused in any single region. It may be more conducive to fitting in the presence of severe burns that cover the regions of traditional weight-bearing (**Fig. 6**). Anticipated activity level may also have an effect on the design of the locations of relative tightness within the socket.[14]

Interface

Given the skin issues discussed, utmost attention is paid to the reduction of shear and slip in the prosthetic socket. Interface stresses between the residual limb and the socket increase significantly when moving from standing to walking and must be accounted for when fitting the prosthesis.[15] The skin will exhibit a thermal response to pressure, but when shear is added the response is increased, although the acceptable level is unknown.[16]

Gel liners are the most common choice of interface for the lower-extremity amputation and have been characterized by their response to compressive, frictional, shear, and tensile loading conditions.[17] Using this information, variations in commercially available gel liners can be matched with patient characteristics to improve the necessary protection between the skin and prosthetic socket. Once a gel liner is chosen, it is

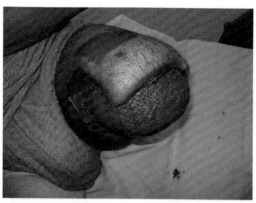

Fig. 6. Compromise of skin integrity over traditional weight-bearing regions of the skin may require the prosthetist to be creative in socket design.

useful to establish the skin tolerance before the prosthetic socket is designed and fabricated. Issues to be aware of include an increased incidence of itching and excess perspiration.[18] The liner can be used as a shrinker if carefully monitored while tolerance is established, although some controversy exists regarding conclusive data related to the functional outcome of gel liner applications compared with other limb-healing modalities.[19,20] Lubrication should be used over bony prominences to reduce the coefficient of friction and allow the liner to slide over these regions during ROM.

When significant limb-shape anomalies are present, some gel liners can be heat-treated over a model of the limb to better conform to the limb and reduce localized pressure in these regions (**Fig. 7**). If heat-treating of a prefabricated liner does not produce the desired contour, a custom-designed liner should be considered. A custom liner can be commercially produced from a digital scan of the limb, with shape and thickness modifications as requested (**Fig. 8**).

Skin problems are associated with the use of prosthetic devices, and therefore diligent hygiene of the skin and liner is of the upmost importance. Commonly reported skin issues associated with prosthetic use include dermatitis, calluses, folliculitis, and ulcerations.[21]

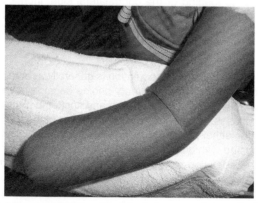

Fig. 7. Prefabricated liner applied to a transradial amputation to facilitate preprosthetic limb-shaping.

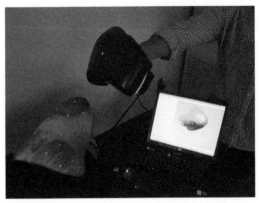

Fig. 8. Some limb shapes will necessitate a fully custom liner fabricated from a digital scan of the residual limb.

Knee

The knee prescription criteria differs little between patients with a burn-related transfemoral amputation and those with nonburn amputations. As in the general transfemoral amputation population, ambulation potential of the patient will determine the appropriate knee classification. Once the socket comfort and skin tolerance are established, the primary concern will be the appropriate knee stability that allows safe use of the limb. Because of the initial cost of the knee component and the multiyear serviceability of today's technology, a prudent approach to prescription is to attempt to determine the ambulation potential of the patient and provide an appropriate knee unit on the first limb that will be usable throughout and even beyond the initial rehabilitation phase.

Because the residual limb is dynamic and will undergo expected size and shape changes, the socket will need periodic replacement, whereas the knee and foot components can remain in use.

One of the most versatile knee units available is the microprocessor controlled unit. This knee can be programmed and adjusted as the patient progresses in ambulation capability, and customized programming options for specific activities can be added (**Fig. 9**). Recent data documenting increased self-selected walking speeds, reduced mental energy, reduced loading of the contralateral side, increased ability for stair descent, cost efficiency, and, perhaps most importantly, a reduced incidence of falls also support its use.[22–27]

Suspension

Suspension of the prosthesis in this population is generally accomplished with one of the suction variations. Suction is the primary choice because it will reduce the incidence of movement between the residual limb and socket in the transitions between swing and stance phases of ambulation. In both transtibial and transfemoral prostheses, suction can be either passive or active. For the transtibial amputation, suction will always be combined with an interface on the limb. Once the limb is placed in the socket, a gel-lined suspension sleeve will be rolled up onto the thigh to create an airtight environment. If suction is passive, a one-way expulsion valve in the distal portion of the socket will allow air to be expelled as the limb is seated into the socket. Once the air is pushed out of the socket, the valve and sleeve prevent air from reentering and the limb is held in proper position, with most piston motion eliminated.

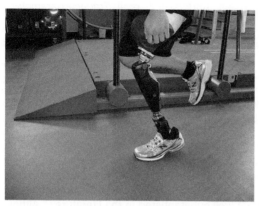

Fig. 9. The many benefits of microprocessor knees include wireless adjustments and the ability for the user to change ambulation modes with a remote control unit.

In an active system, the air is removed from the socket with a mechanical or electronic pump. In some systems, the vacuum level can be set and the pump will maintain the vacuum at the predetermined status. Vacuum is reported to help control volume fluctuations, reduce piston motion of the residual limb, and provide a secure feeling of attachment between the limb and the prosthesis (**Fig. 10**).

If a vacuum system is not indicated and the desire is to allow increased range about the knee, a pin system can be used. A pin suspension still uses a gel interface, but

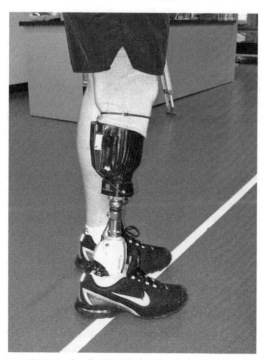

Fig. 10. Vacuum suspension can be facilitated by the use of an electric pump that is activated by the user.

instead of suction, a pin is attached to a receptacle at the distal end of the liner and will be locked into the distal end of the prosthesis when donned. This eliminates the need for a suspension sleeve but may not feel as secure as a suction system.

Foot/Ankle

Foot and ankle choices are not specific to the burn population. As with the knee options, feet should be prescribed with the activity level and ambulation potential in mind. Unlike prosthetic knees, feet are manufactured for specific weight ranges. Most feet have approximately a 30-lb weight range. If the patient has weight gain or loss that moves them out of the prescribed category, the foot will need to be changed for comfortable ambulation to continue. Energy storage and return (ESAR) feet are the most commonly recommended prosthesis for the active population and most often requested by patients, even though significant reduction in energy cost or enhanced prosthetic gait are not well substantiated in the literature.[28] Although a more flexible foot may be most beneficial in protecting the residual limb, one double-blind study showed that most patients preferred a less-flexible foot.[29] Different ESAR foot designs affect the amount of compliance of the device. This compliance or flexibility difference will affect changes in patient muscle activity and measureable energy return. Careful attention to foot stiffness can improve rehabilitation outcomes.[30]

Components in the shank that will allow transverse rotation can be added to reduce shear stress on the residual limb during stance phase. These components have been shown to reduce prosthetic–limb peak internal rotation moments when walking in a circular motion.[31] Reduction of this motion can reduce the skin stresses that occur between the socket and limb. Although some patients may find this rotation gives them a feeling of instability, it should still be considered and even tried on trial basis for most burn patients, and especially those with bilateral amputations.[32]

Alignment

One last factor in the design of the prosthesis is alignment. Regardless of the amputation level, the alignment relationships among the socket, knee, ankle, and foot are critical in efficient ambulation and force applications on the residual limb. In the transfemoral amputation, sagittal alignment has a direct correlation to knee stability. The more posterior the knee is in relation to the socket and ankle, the more stable it will be in the stance phase of gait. This stability, however, will come at the cost of decreased energy efficiency, because the patient will need to use increased hip flexion power to initiate knee flexion.

More critical to the burn patient is how alignment will affect the pressures on the residual limb in the sagittal and coronal planes (**Fig. 11**). Changes in alignment will affect the joint moments, which will change the corresponding pressures that occur at specific regions of the limb. Testing force couples on the limb during evaluation and paying particular attention to regions of the limb that must accept these pressures will help protect the skin from undue pressure and shear. If alignment is used to unload areas of the limb, then one must understand that gait anomalies may result. The clinical team will need to find the balance between skin protection and gait efficiency.

UPPER-EXTREMITY PROSTHETIC DESIGN CONSIDERATIONS

Considerations regarding socket design and fabrication and the type of prosthetic control system, suspension, wrist, and terminal devices are paramount when addressing range of motion limitations and maximizing optimal function to facilitate patient independence with the prosthesis (**Fig. 12**). In the authors' experience, the design

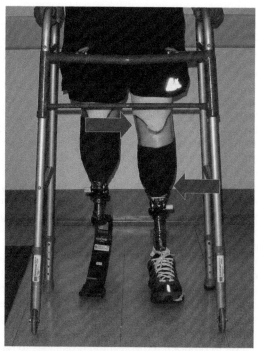

Fig. 11. Careful attention must be paid to how the alignment will affect the pressures applied to the residual limb during ambulation (*arrows*).

of the upper-extremity prosthesis must allow for self-care, such as toileting, eating, driving, and using a cell phone. If the prosthesis does not allow independence in performing these activities, patients will find ways to accomplish those tasks without a prosthesis, even those who have a bilaterally involved upper-extremity amputation.

Although independence without a prosthesis is helpful, patients have experienced a disservice if a caregiver is needed only because of the inadequacy of the prosthetic device. This independence begins with the ability to don and doff the limb.

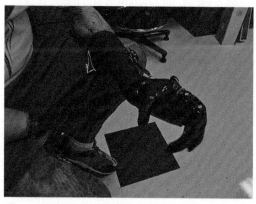

Fig. 12. A mechanically operated partial hand prosthesis aids in functional independence in this bilateral patient.

Problem-solving the donning and doffing methods may be achieved through discussions and trial and error among the patient, prosthetist, and occupational therapist.

Limitations in range of motion also influence the decision process regarding the type of prostheses best suited for the patient. A conventional or even hybrid cable-operated prosthesis requires significant range of motion at the shoulder and glenohumeral joint for both the affected and contralateral side. Although conventional or body powered prostheses are commonly prescribed first because of cost saving attempts, amputations that involve burned and grafted skin or grafted skin covering the proximal intact joints may be most successfully fitted as a myoelectric system.

In many cases, the harness control system of a body-powered limb can be abrasive and very uncomfortable, and can limit the available range of motion that is already compromised because of issues such as heterotrophic ossification and skin adhesions. Although very costly as an initial modality, a full myoelectric system can provide greater range of motion of the intact limb and more efficient range of motion of a myoelectric elbow or wrist. The patient's range of motion may gradually increase and the integrity of the skin may improve enough to allow a conventional or body-powered prosthesis to be operated without difficulty.

As the initial prescription is developed, the cognitive load associated with complicated control systems must be considered. Each aspect of the prosthesis can subject patients to an increased level of thought required to properly use and operate the device as designed. A balance must be sought that allows patients to experience optimal functionality and an overall sense of success. If the cognitive load is too great, the potential for various types of functional failures may increase. One example of reducing the cognitive load would be to program a myoelectric prosthesis to have standard hand open-and-close signals but to keep the wrist unit powered off until the patient masters isolated hand function, at which time the wrist unit can be powered on and programmed to allow the patient a stepwise progression in the rehabilitation process. Setting reasonable goals with incorporation of activities and prosthetic technology allows patients to experience small victories and accomplishments during the rehabilitation process, keeping them engaged and encouraged by their accomplishments.

As the first prosthesis is designed, all involved parties must understand that it is simply the initial test system. This initial prosthesis is a starting point from which to build and learn for both patients and caregivers. This process may show that the initial test system is the best for the patient in the long term. Some of the early discussion points can be as simple as the type and location of the power switch, socket alignment angles, terminal devices choices, programming and mode of operation, and even the entire socket design. The test system is usually fabricated with temporary heat-moldable plastics to allow for adjustment of volume changes, pressure distribution, limb length, and functional socket angles. The arm is designed to be used in therapy and outside the facility in real-world situations.

Amputation Level Determination

The decision-making process regarding amputation level may vary greatly among treatment centers. Past experience and training of the surgeons, prosthetists, physical medicine physicians, and therapists will play a role in this process. For example, various socket designs are now available that may make a wrist disarticulation design preferred over a transradial design, especially when the skin around the elbow may not tolerate the necessary proximal forces and higher proximal trimlines of the transradial socket system. The wrist disarticulation may also prove useful if the patient has sustained bilateral amputations. Donning a wrist disarticulation prosthesis may be more efficient and easier for them as a bilateral amputee, particularly when the other side is transradial or higher. Although it initially sounds counterintuitive, a shoulder disarticulation may even be preferred over a short transhumeral socket if the patient has significant glenohumeral range of motion restrictions that are expected to limit their ability to use a prosthesis. A more proximal amputation may also be considered if electromyogram signals are unobtainable at a lower level.

Socket and Interface Design

The socket system is the foundation for control of the entire prosthesis. Compromised surface tissues must somehow now interface with various synthetic materials and incur levels of shear, slip, torque, pressure, and distraction all amplified by the weight of the arm itself. The most common choices of interface include prefabricated roll-on liners, custom-designed roll-on liners, direct socket interfacing, or even custom static inner silicon liners. Each of these has the potential to work, but the decision is again made on an individual basis and is influenced by past experience of the prosthetist and other members of the team. For example, the prefabricated liners range in elasticity, coefficient of friction, and material, all of which must be matched with the limb characteristics.

A direct socket interface without a custom liner is also a viable option. In the authors' experience, this custom-molded liner is fabricated using low durometer silicone that can also incorporate the electrodes if a myoelectric system is desired. The custom static silicon inner liner is fabricated using materials that most closely mimic the elasticity and integrity of normal skin and tissue. This material works very well in cases of delayed healing and tenuous tissue, with or without the use of light friction-reducing dressings on the limb. It can also accommodate moderate levels of limb volume fluctuation and reduce the difficulty of donning the prosthesis over irregular shapes and compromised or even open skin. The socket system is donned using readily available lubricants. This custom interface can even be used as a shrinker before full fabrication of the socket (**Fig. 13**).

When completed, this liner is fixated within the structural frame of the socket and the additional components are attached.

Once the appropriate inner socket interface is provided, the outer structural shell and socket is begun. The outer socket will provide the structural integrity necessary to properly transmit forces from the limb to the prosthesis, and provide an attachment

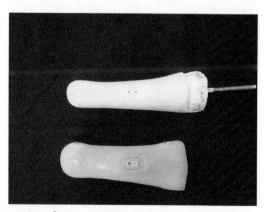

Fig. 13. Custom silicone interfaces are used to facilitate wound healing, accommodate irregular shapes, and provide limb volume control. Shown are both the liner and mold of the patient limb.

basis for the other prosthetic components. Rotational control of the prosthesis is a significant problem that can be addressed in two ways. The use of significantly higher proximal trimlines may be necessary to add control of the prosthesis on the more proximal amputations. Rotational control must also be addressed within the body of the socket through careful design of pressures that will compress and displace the soft tissue in relationship to the bony anatomy.

Most of the socket stability should come from the design of the contours that place pressure on the tolerant areas of the limb, and then secondarily through suspension sleeves and harnessing designs. These load-bearing regions must be very well thought out. The obvious unloading of bony anatomy is required, but with burned and grafted tissue, high focal pressures may result in undesired skin breakdown. Often little underlying subcutaneous tissue is available to protect underling muscle and tendons. If myoelectric control is desired, design consideration must be given to prevent excess pressure that can degrade the thin skin and develop into a skin ulcer at the myosite.

Suspension

Suspension of the prosthesis can come in a single form or multiple forms working together (**Fig. 14**). In general, the prosthesis should be suspended using as much skin surface area as possible. Focalized suspension, as in the case with pin locking and sealing ring liners, may be prone to exhibit increased levels of skin friction over tenuous or fragile skin because of the distally located suspension mechanisms of these systems. Full-contact suction using a static custom silicone liner can be applied at the partial hand, wrist disarticulation, transradial, elbow disarticulation, and

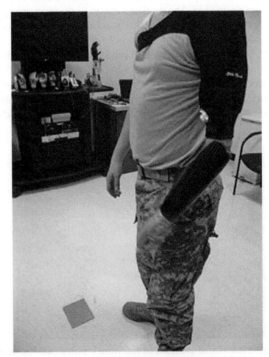

Fig. 14. Full myoelectric transhumeral prosthesis suspended with suction and an auxiliary neoprene suspension harness.

transhumeral levels. This system provides suction suspension over the length of the limb yet protects the skin with the pliable silicone.

In some cases, use of just skin suction can provide even greater levels of suspension and the active volume control commonly seen in the lower-extremity prosthetic design. This design uses no interface between the residual limb and socket but relies only on skin tension and an airtight control of the limb volume. This method gives the most direct control and proprioceptive control of the prosthesis. Although it does require sensate, elastic skin, it can be appropriate for this population in isolated incidences. As with any active suction system, the potential for acute tissue damage increases with factors such as lack of patient awareness of changes in limb volume, high level of complexity of proper donning of the prosthesis, and improper activation of the vacuum system.

In addition to various forms of suction, variations in socket shape may help suspension over bony anatomy. Most commonly, this is achieved through capturing the styloids in the wrist disarticulation and humeral epicondyles in both the transradial and elbow disarticulation applications. In addition to suspension, capture of this anatomy can also provide substantial rotational control of the socket. Although use of this form of suspension is vital to adequate prosthetic suspension and control, the degree to which it is used will depend on the tissue tolerance of the skin in these regions.

Harnessing is a form of suspension that can also be used as a control mechanism if the prosthesis is designed to be body-powered. In most myoelectric prostheses at the transradial and wrist disarticulation levels, the sockets do not need to be adequately self-suspended by suction. The goal of harnessing is to use it only when needed and with specific purpose. If the prosthesis has maximized function, control, and suspension, a harness is not required. If a prosthetic system can be designed that has minimal to no harness, patients will greatly benefit from increased range of motion and freedom of movement, and generalized increased levels of comfort. If function, control, and suspension are not optimal with an existing system of any level, then harnessing is required or an existing harness must be modified to achieve the desired function. However, if harnessing is relied on too much for function, control, or suspension, then the socket design and suspension will most likely require significant changes to improve those areas.

Elbow Options

With amputations at or above the elbow, several variations exist in prosthetic elbow choices. The body-powered elbow systems require a significant amount of scapular and glenohumeral range of motion for full use. Various combinations of shoulder motion are captured by the harness system to produce combinations of elbow flexion, terminal device operation, and positional elbow locking. A fully body-powered system requires the greatest shoulder range for operation of both the mechanical elbow and terminal device operation. Although a mechanical elbow may require the largest degree of strength and range, it is also places the least cognitive load on the patient. This body-powered elbow is the most commonly prescribed prosthetic elbow for a new prosthetic user, such as a person with a recent amputation or one who has not previously chosen to use a prosthesis. A common approach is to prescribe a conventional body-powered above-elbow prosthesis to begin the rehabilitation process and establish a prosthetic use pattern.

Once the patient demonstrates successful use of this simple prosthetic design, a hybrid or fully electronic prosthetic system may be considered. This approach is reasonable as long as a body-powered system is still the right choice. If other limitations to using harnessing and body power exist, use of a conventional prosthesis will likely not be successful and the patient could reject any use of a prosthetic device.

When physical limitations exist in implementing body power, a hybrid design should be considered. A hybrid system most commonly includes a mechanical elbow with a myoelectric hand and wrist rotator. The hybrid prosthetic system uses a traditional harness for body-powered activation of elbow movement in combination an electronically operated wrist and terminal device function. The terminal device and wrist can be electromyogram- or mechanical switch–controlled. The compromise in introducing electronics includes an increased level of cognitive load and associated training, moderate increase in weight associated with the electronic wrist, terminal device and battery, and significant cost increase.

If appropriate, a fully electronic system can be provided that includes electronic function of all aspects of the prosthesis, including the elbow, wrist, and hand. It may operated with use of one to two electrodes and other electronically activated pull switches, force sensors, or cable tension–activated transducers (**Fig. 15**). The fully electronic above-elbow prosthesis requires the least amount of harness-activated movement and shoulder range of motion to perform the desired function. This system is the heaviest and most costly. In the burn amputation population, the traditional mindset of demonstrating mastery of a body-powered prosthesis before considering electronics may not actually be in the best interest of the patient for several reasons. The shear forces across the burned skin and grafted tissue caused by body-powered harness systems is rarely tolerated within the first 3 to 6 months of prosthetic use. Many of these patients do not have adequate range of motion or ability to generate joint power to operate a conventional or hybrid elbow system. In the absence of joint range and strength, they may still be able to operate a fully electronic elbow system

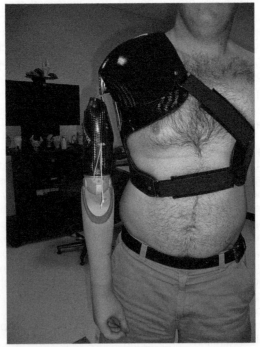

Fig. 15. Fully myoelectric control is provided in this shoulder disarticulation prosthesis.

with electromyogram activation or another form of electronic operation of the elbow, wrist, and hand.

If this system is chosen, careful attention must be given to appropriate socket design, skin interface, and the secondary suspension harness that will enable the patient to tolerate use of a complicated, heavy limb. Many of these elbow systems allow for gradual progression of function in the early phases of rehabilitation and training through incorporating wireless programming options through an on-board microprocessor. This gradual progression of the complexity of the system allows for reduced cognitive load in early training and advancement of the elbow function when appropriate.

One additional challenge to be aware of is the effect of the elbow choice on limb length and matching anatomic elbow centers. The elbow disarticulation amputation has limited elbow options. Although it can be a very functional level, it will require the use of mechanical outside locking hinges to keep bilateral elbow centers equal and maintain some symmetry in appearance to the sound side. Outside locking hinges can be used in either a conventional body-powered prosthesis or even the hybrid version, depending on the patients needs. Although generally not cosmetically acceptable, a fully electronic above-elbow system may be warranted to enable optimized levels of function and independence from limited range of motion and levels of skin integrity. Occasionally, if extended wheelchair use is necessary because of lower-extremity complications, a powered system may be necessary overcome the limitations of using body power while seated.

Wrist and Hand Options

In this patient population, normal joint range of motion is rarely seen. Furthermore, it is common to encounter bilateral upper extremity involvement in which the sound contralateral side has amputation or is intact but has compromised strength and range in the hand, wrist, elbow, or shoulder. Given this scenario, the choice of terminal device and wrist unit are even more important.

A primary goal with any prosthesis, whether body-powered or myoelectric, is to enable patients to reach midline for eating and toileting purposes (**Fig. 16**). How this basic fundamental principle is achieved does not really matter, but plenty of options are available to the well-informed treatment team. Although other tasks that facilitate

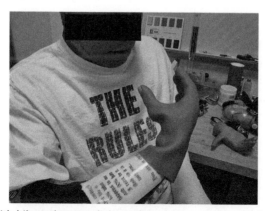

Fig. 16. Patient with bilateral transradial prostheses demonstrating limited neck, shoulder, and elbow range of motion.

independence are also important, these are milestones of the early rehabilitation goals.

Terminal devices will be manually or electrically controlled. The goal is to select a mechanical or myoelectric terminal device and wrist combination that allows for the greatest function to facilitate activities of daily living. Minimal advances in technology regarding the mechanically operated terminal device and wrist have been made, but they remain a standard of care because of affordability and durability. The standard conventional options include the traditional opening and closing devices that are hand- or hook-based and offer various locking mechanism for a sure grip on an item (**Fig. 17**). Wrist flexion systems are also available that are a separate component or may be integrated into the terminal device. A few cable-operated mechanical wrist rotation systems are produced, but their use and function are limited.

If a myoelectric device is desired, one must overcome the challenge of gaining access to these advanced systems. They require specialized skill by the provider and will incur significant cost that must be justified to the payor. Although not for everyone, their benefits are numerous. As in many of the elbow and knee systems, the terminal devices have microprocessor control and blue tooth programmability. The prosthesis and associated terminal device can be configured to best meet the needs of the patient with real-time adjustments of electromyogram gain and thresholds, speed, grip force, and control patterns. One of the most significant advances is the option to have multiple gasp pattern choices on a single myoelectric hand system. This function has allowed patients to expand the grip options with a simple control sequence that can be performed in less than a second. Some of these additional patterns can include pinch grasp, three jaw chuck, lateral pinch, and power grip. In addition to these current advances in technology, various forms of electronic wrist flexion and extension and ulnar and radial deviation will be available soon.

With advances in the electronic hardware for the upper extremity, the methods of purposeful control become more complicated (**Fig. 18**).

There is a significant focus on research related to developing proprioceptive feedback and neural interface through the surgical modification of nerves such as targeted muscle reinnervation, electromyogram implants, cortical implants, and pattern grasp recognition.[33,34]

However, no perfect terminal device or control strategy exists that will facilitate every activity. When feasible, it is best to allow patients to trial multiple terminal devices outside of the clinical setting; this will help them develop an understanding

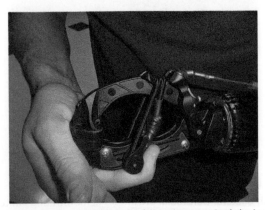

Fig. 17. Body-powered, voluntary opening, multitension terminal device.

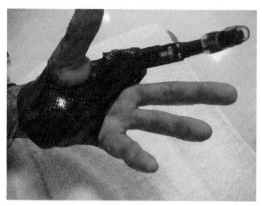

Fig. 18. Myoelectric control of a partial hand prosthesis is shown in this single-digit device.

of the capability of each, and how a particular device may be best suited to their needs.

As is continually experienced with lower-extremity prosthetic advances, access to this technology must be supported by evidence of the outcome benefits, or request for insurance coverage will usually be denied. Given the smaller sample size of the individuals with upper-extremity amputation, completing large functional trials will continue to be challenging.

Follow-up and Long-Term Care

When patients are nearing completion of their formal rehabilitation, they will need to be educated on the importance of self-advocacy. If they were treated at a burn treatment center, they probably were care for by a highly skilled treatment team very familiar with the burn rehabilitation process. Once patients complete therapy and are discharged from care, the need for a skilled prosthetist remains. The socket will need to be replaced as the limb undergoes expected changes, and the powered components will need service and adjustment. If the patients were provided and trained with a complex powered system, they may experience difficulty having service and maintenance performed in their local community. It is prudent to consider providing patients with a simple backup system to be used in the inevitable situation when the complex powered limb needs service, and providing simple customized assistive devices for optimal performance of daily activities.[35,36]

SUMMARY

Technology is ever-changing and it is daunting to try and keep up with all of the advances in upper- and lower-extremity prosthetics. Teams treating patients with complex burn amputations must continue sharing the advances made within each of their scopes of practice. These practice lines can become blurred depending on the treatment philosophy of the center and availability of each discipline. However, having a working knowledge of each of the disciplines involved will always be in the patient's best interest. The future for prosthetics and associated advances is very promising, but the goal for these systems is not the same for every patient. Clinical professionals must be willing to provide patients with technology and training in a systematic yet very flexible manner; this will enable the entire process to be tailored to best meet the usually complicated individual needs of patients with burn-related limb loss.

REFERENCES

1. Ward RS, Hayes-Lundy C, Schnebly WA, et al. Prosthetic use in patients with burns and associated limb amputations. J Burn Care Rehabil 1990;11(4):361–4.
2. Kennedy PJ, Young WM, Deva AK, et al. Burns and amputations: a 24-year experience. J Burn Care Res 2006;27(2):183–8.
3. Luz DP, Millan LS, Alessi MS, et al. Electrical burns: a retrospective analysis across a 5 year period. Burns 2009;35(7):1015–9.
4. Pannucci CJ, Osborne NH, Jaber RM, et al. Early fasciotomy in electrically injured patients as a marker for injury severity and deep venous thrombosis risk: an analysis of the national burn repository. J Burn Care Res 2010;31(6):882–7.
5. Hedawoo JB, Ali A. Electric burns and disability. J Indian Med Assoc 2010; 108(2):84–7.
6. Herrera FA, Hassanein AH, Potenza B, et al. Bilateral upper extremity vascular injury as a result of a high voltage electrical burn. Ann Vasc Surg 2010;24(6): 825.e1–5.
7. Baumeister S, Koller M, Dragu A, et al. Principles of microvascular reconstruction in burn and electrical burn injuries. Burns 2005;31(1):92–8.
8. Yowler CJ, Mozingo DW, Ryan JB, et al. Factors contributing to delayed extremity amputation in burn patients. J Trauma 1998;45(3):522–6.
9. Schneider JF, Holavanahalli R, Helm P, et al. Contractures in burn injury: defining the problem. J Burn Care Res 2006;27(4):508–14.
10. Chen MC, Lee SS, Hsieh YL, et al. Influencing factors of outcome after lower limb amputation: a five year review in a plastic surgical department. Ann Plast Surg 2008;61(3):314–8.
11. Fergason J, Smith DG. Socket considerations for the patient with a transtibial amputation. Clin Orthop Relat Res 1999;(361):76–84.
12. Yowler CJ, Patterson BM, Brandt CP, et al. Osteocutaneous pedicle flap of the foot for salvage of below-knee amputation level after burn injury. J Burn Care Rehabil 2001;22(1):21–5.
13. Acikel C, Peker F, Akmaz I, et al. Muscle transposition and skin grafting for salvage of below knee amputation level after bilateral lower extremity thermal injury. Burns 2001;27(8):849–52.
14. Isozaki K, Hosoda M, Masuda T, et al. CAD/DAM evaluation of the fit of trans-tibial amputation stumps. J Med Dent Sci 2006;53(1):51–6.
15. Zachariah SG, Sanders JE. Standing interface stresses as predictor of walking interface stresses in the trans-tibial prosthesis. Prosthet Orthot Int 2001;25(1): 34–40.
16. Sanders JE. Thermal response of skin to cyclic pressure and pressure with shear: a technical note. J Rehabil Res Dev 2000;37(5):511–5.
17. Sanders JE, Nicholson BS, Zachariah SG, et al. Testing of elastomeric liners used in limb prosthetics: classification of 15 products by mechanical performance. J Rehabil Res Dev 2004;41(2):175–86.
18. Baars EC, Geertzen JH. Literature review of the possible advantages of silicon liner socket use in transtibial prostheses. Prosthet Orthot Int 2005;29(1):27–37.
19. Nawijn SE, Van der Linde H, Emmelot CH, et al. Stump management after trans-tibial amputation: a systematic review. Prosthet Orthot Int 2005;29(1): 13–26.
20. Van Velzen AD, Nederhand MJ, Emmelot CH, et al. Early treatment of transtibial amputees: retrospective analysis of early fitting and elastic bandaging. Prosthet Orthot Int 2005;29(1):3–12.

21. Almass F, Mousavi B, Masumi M, et al. Skin disorders associated with bilateral lower extremity amputation. Pak J Biol Sci 2009;12(20):1381–4.
22. Bellmann M, Schmalz T, Blumentritt S. Comparative biomechanical analysis of current microprocessor-controlled prosthetic knee joints. Arch Phys Med Rehabil 2010;91(4):644–52.
23. Maaref K, Martinet N, Grumillier C, et al. Kinematics in the terminal swing phase of unilateral transfemoral amputees: microprocessor-controlled versus swing-phase control prosthetic knees. Arch Phys Med Rehabil 2010;91(6):919–25.
24. Hafner BJ, Smith DG. Differences in function and safety between Medicare Functional Classification Level-2 and -3 transfemoral amputees and influence of prosthetic knee joint control. J Rehabil Res Dev 2009;46(3):417–33.
25. Kahle JT, Highsmith MJ, Hubbard SL. Comparison of nonmicroprocessor knee mechanism versus C-leg on Prosthesis Evaluation Questionnaire, stumbles, falls, walking tests, stair descent, and knee preference. J Rehabil Res Dev 2008;45(1): 1–14.
26. Broadkorb TH, Henriksson M, Johannesen-Muck K, et al. Cost-effectiveness of C-Leg compared with non-microprocessor-controlled knees: a modeling approach. Arch Phys Med Rehabil 2008;89(1):24–30.
27. Aufman KR, Levine JA, Brey RH, et al. Energy expenditure and activity of transfemoral amputees using mechanical and microprocessor-controlled prosthetic knees. Arch Phys Med Rehabil 2008;89(7):1380–5.
28. Versluys R, Beyl P, Van Damme M, et al. Prosthetic feet: state-of-the-art review and the importance of mimicking human ankle-foot biomechanics. Disabil Rehabil Assist Technol 2009;4(2):65–75.
29. Klodd E, Hansen A, Fatone S, et al. Effects of prosthetic foot forefoot flexibility on oxygen cost and subjective preference rankings of unilateral transtibial prosthesis users. J Rehabil Res Dev 2010;47(6):543–52.
30. Ventura JD, Klute GK, Neptune RR. The effect of prosthetic ankle energy storage and return properties on muscle activity in below-knee amputee walking. Gait Posture 2011;33(2):220–6.
31. Segal AD, Orendurff MS, Czerniecki JM, et al. Transtibial amputee joint rotation moments during straight-line walking and a common turning task with and without torsion adapter. J Rehabil Res Dev 2009;46(3):375–83.
32. Su PF, Gard SA, Lipschutz RD, et al. The effects of increased prosthetic ankle motions on the gait of persons with bilateral transtibial amputations. Am J Phys Med Rehabil 2010;89(1):34–47.
33. Farrell TR, Weir RF, Heckathorn CW, et al. The effects of static friction and backlash on extended physiological proprioception control of a powered prosthesis. J Rehabil Res Dev 2005;42(3):327–41.
34. Dhillon GS, Horch KW. Direct neural sensory feedback and control of a prosthetic arm. IEEE Trans Neural Syst Rehabil Eng 2005;13(4):468–72.
35. Chang JK. Assistive devices in the rehabilitation on patients with electrical burns—three case reports. J Burn Care Rehabil 2001;22(1):90–6.
36. Hung JW, Wu YH. Fitting a bilateral transhumeral amputee wit utensil prostheses and their functional assessment 10 years later: a case report. Arch Phys Med Rehabil 2005;86(11):2211–3.

Hypertrophic Scar

Vincent Gabriel, MD, MSc, FRCPC[a,b,*]

KEYWORDS

- Hypertrophic scar • Wound healing • Keloids
- Rehabilitation • Scar measurement

Hypertrophic burn scars are the most common complication of burn injury.[1] Although the worldwide prevalence of hypertrophic scars is not known, it is estimated that up to 1 million burn injuries occur annually in the United States. This may represent a small portion of the worldwide burden of burns and scarring as the incidence of burn injury is much higher in underdeveloped countries.[2] Hypertrophic scars may be seen after other soft tissue injuries, including surgical incisions, compound fractures, or other wounds.

In a 10-year review of burn injury admissions in North America, approximately 95% of patients survived their hospital stays.[3] This impressive survival rate means that a great number of patients bear the life-long burden of hypertrophic scars.

STAGES OF WOUND HEALING AND THE WOUND HEALING SPECTRUM

Under normal circumstances wound healing progresses in an orderly fashion. Normal wound healing may be divided in to inflammatory, proliferative, and remodeling phases. In the inflammatory phase, the injury and resultant cellular debris initiate platelet aggregation and the migration of leukocytes and macrophages to the wound site. The clot that develops to create a seal of the wound serves as a matrix for promoting further cellular migration into the wound bed.

I have no significant financial conflicts of interest with the material in this document.

Support for some of the content in this manuscript comes from National Center for Medical Rehabilitation Research at the National Institute of Child Health and Human Development, National Institutes of Health, and the Association of Academic Physiatrists (K12 HD1001097–13) and National Institute for Disability and Rehabilitation Research Office of Special Education and Rehabilitative Services, US Department of Education (H133A20104).

Written consent for all photography is stored in the Department of Physical Medicine and Rehabilitation, UT SW, 5161 Harry Hines Boulevard, Dallas, TX 75390–9055. None of the figures included have been submitted for publication in another manuscript.

[a] Division of Physical Medicine and Rehabilitation, Fire Fighters Burn Treatment Centre, Foothills Medical Centre, University of Calgary, 1403-29 Street NW, Calgary, Alberta T2N 2T9, Canada

[b] Division of Physical Medicine and Rehabilitation, Department of Clinical Neurosciences, Foothills Medical Centre, Room AW 122-Foothills Hospital, 1403–29 Street NW, Calgary, Alberta T2N 2T9, Canada

* Division of Physical Medicine and Rehabilitation, Department of Clinical Neurosciences, Foothills Medical Centre, Room AW 122-Foothills Hospital, 1403–29 Street NW, Calgary, Alberta T2N 2T9, Canada.

E-mail address: vincent.gabriel@ualberta.ca

Phys Med Rehabil Clin N Am 22 (2011) 301–310

doi:10.1016/j.pmr.2011.02.002

pmr.theclinics.com

1047-9651/11/$ – see front matter © 2011 Elsevier Inc. All rights reserved.

Approximately 3 days after the initial injury, at the start of the proliferative phase, other cell types are activated to enter the wound such as fibroblasts and vascular cells. After approximately 5 days after injury, epidermal cells begin to proliferate and migrate over the surface of the wound and the provisional matrix below.

Through the remodeling phase over the course of the following weeks and even months, further changes occur in the wound as the collagen deposition by local fibroblasts changes to have a predominance of type 1 over type 3 collagen and the vascular structures mature.[4]

The desirable result of normal wound healing is replacement of the initial hemostatic clot with skin that approximates the aesthetic, mechanical, and functional properties of the preinjury tissue. Changes in the steps of normal wound healing may result in either a "hypoplastic" or chronic nonhealing wound or the hypertrophic "over-healed" wound.

Many clinicians are familiar with the "under-healed" chronic wound. Impediments to normal wound healing may include intrinsic metabolic abnormalities such as vascular diseases or diabetes. The nonhealing chronic wound may be exacerbated by extrinsic biologic factors such as the presence of bioburden as well as extrinsic mechanical factors such as excessive pressure in patients with impaired sensation, sensorium, or motor function.[5–7]

The opposite end of the wound healing spectrum are the dermatoproliferative disorders: hypertrophic and keloid scarring. Hypertrophic scars differ clinically from keloid scars in that hypertrophic scars are described as developing within the margins of the original injury, whereas keloid scars may extend beyond the original injury.[8,9] Hypertrophic scars are described as raised from the surrounding skin. They are painful, pruritic, and contractile.[9] A comparison of the spectrum of clinical outcomes in wound healing is made in **Table 1**.

RISK FACTORS FOR DEVELOPMENT OF HYPERTROPHIC SCARS

Although there have been advances in developing technology to predict healing in burn wounds, there are no reliable tools presently available to predict which wounds will develop in to hypertrophic burn scars.[10] Clinical experience suggests that patients whom have darker pigmented skin are more likely to develop a dermatoproliferative disorder. Also, adolescents are thought to have a higher likelihood of developing

Table 1
Spectrum of wound healing

Result	Chronic Nonhealing Wound Ulcer	Normal Healing	Dermatoproliferative Disorders
Clinical Characteristics	Exudating, nonepithelialized	Epithelialized, approximates preinjury functional properties, and is aesthetically and mechanically acceptable	Epithelialized, increased volume, erythema, contracture, pruritus, chronic dynamic process of inflammation and fibrosis
Factors	Inadequate substrates, excessive mechanical forces, excessive moisture, bioburden	Appropriate substrates, vascularity, minimization of mechanical forces and bioburden, moist wound-healing environment	Prolonged inflammatory wound healing phase, activated transforming growth factor-beta signaling

a hypertrophic scar than adults.[9] The best clinical predictor for the development of hypertrophic burn scars is a prolonged inflammatory wound healing phase. This would usually correspond with a wound that has not epithelialized and continues to exudate for more than 3 weeks.[11]

Burn wound depths are described as superficial, partial thickness, or full thickness. Superficial burns, such as sunburn can be expected to heal spontaneously in approximately 10 days without a significant risk of hypertrophic scarring. Superficial partial-thickness burns such as a typical household scald injury result in blistering, painful wounds that should be expected to epithelialize within approximately 2 weeks provided no complications arise in the wound healing process. The risk of developing hypertrophic burn scars from superficial partial-thickness buns is low, but not zero.

Deep partial-thickness burns have less blistering than superficial partial-thickness burns, are painful, and may take up to 3 weeks or longer to epithelialize. The risk of scarring with deep partial-thickness burns is significant. Full-thickness burns destroy the epidermis and dermis and result in burn wounds that may be less painful than partial-thickness burns and typically have limited exudate but may present with necrotic eschar. The risk of hypertrophic scarring from full-thickness burns is high.

Different anatomic regions seem to have different risks for the development of hypertrophic scars. For example, it is unusual to observe the development of hypertrophic scars on the scalp, eyelid, or palm of the hand.[11]

CELLULAR SIGNALS AND PATHWAYS IN HYPERTROPHIC SCARRING

Several cellular signals are implicated as having an important role in the development of hypertrophic scars. One signal thought to be of particular importance is transforming growth factor-beta (TGF-β). This protein is part of a large family including bone morphogenic proteins and activins. TGF-β exists in both latent and activated forms. TGF-β acts through a signaling pathway mediated by the SMAD proteins. The net effect of activated TGF-β interacting with the TGF-β receptor and activation of the SMAD pathway in fibroblasts appears to be an increase in production of extracellular matrix and signals leading to cellular proliferation.[12,13] Over time, some cells can develop autocrine TGF-β positive feedback loops that can lead to a self-propagating cycle of excessive extracellular matrix production and cell proliferation.[14]

Hypertrophic scars are dynamic and express different histologic appearances, cellular signals, and molecular characteristics depending on the stage of development. This may result in conflicting descriptions of the microscopic hypertrophic scar environment.[15]

Excessive extracellular matrix formation does not account for all of the clinical characteristics of hypertrophic scars. Overall, an imbalance between too much matrix formation and inadequate matrix remodeling is thought to exist as the overall milieu in hypertrophic scarring. Cellular signaling between keratinocytes and fibroblasts is an important component of this process and there is some evidence that keratinocyte signals such as stratifin may activate matrix metalloproteinases that would have an important effect on scar fibroblasts in reorganizing extracellular matrix proteins.[16] Multiple other cell types, including mast cells and bone-marrow–derived mesenchymal stem cells, are also present in the hypertrophic scar and are likely significant in clinical characteristics of the hypertrophic scarring phenotype.[12]

CLINICAL CHARACTERISTICS AND MEASUREMENT OF HYPERTROPHIC SCARS

Hypertrophic burn scars develop during the remodeling phase of wound healing, typically in the first few months of injury. During this time, the volume increases and the scars become contractile and erythematous. However, after several months, the scars may show spontaneous regression without complete resolution to normal skin. **Fig. 1** shows a hypertrophic scar on the shoulder of a patient 20 months after original injury.[9] This patient was injured with scalding water at 13-months-old.

Although hypertrophic burn scars may show regression, there is significant heterogeneity in the volume, erythema, and pigmentation within a single scar, as shown in **Fig. 2**. In this case, the photograph was taken 21 months after deep partial-thickness flame burns. The peripheral margins of the scars have regressed in volume and erythema; however, the texture and volume of the scars in the left flank and arm are significantly abnormal compared with the surrounding skin.

The description of hypertrophic burn scars therefore poses a challenge to the rehabilitation practitioner. There are several clinical tools used to try to describe hypertrophic scars. The Vancouver Scar Scale (VSS) is a clinician rating scale that includes items to describe vascularity, height, pliability, and pigmentation in a scar. With the Patient and Observer Scar Assessment Scale, an observer rates the scar on vascularity, thickness, relief, pliability, surface area, and pliability while a patient assesses color, stiffness, thickness, relief, and itching. The Manchester Scale assesses color as compared with surrounding normal skin for appearance, contour, texture, size, number, and characteristics of the margins or borders of the scar.[17] Overall, the VSS is probably the most widely used and applicable to the burn scar patient.[18]

However, there are several limitations in using the VSS. In a large scar, such as the one in **Fig. 2**, it can be unclear which area of the scar the VSS is being used to rate. Also, because it is a subjective rating scale, it may not accurately describe characteristics such as volume.[19]

An ideal measurement tool for the description of a hypertrophic burn scar would be valid, reliable, sensitive to change over time, and include characteristics such as volume, viscoelastic properties, and color.

The viscoelastic or biomechanical properties of skin and scar may be measured with a device known as a Cutometer (Courage + Khazaka electronic GmbH, Köln, Germany). These devices measure deformation in the skin or scar by the application of a vacuum chamber and measurement of laser light reflectance. With a known

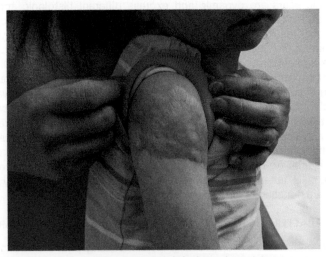

Fig. 1. Hypertrophic burn scar following partial-thickness burn injury.

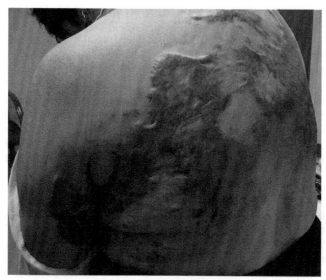

Fig. 2. Heterogeneity of hypertrophic burn scar with peripheral regression but ongoing active scarring in the periscapular regions, left flank, and left arm.

vacuum force and quantifiable deformation in the skin or scar, calculations may be made for descriptors of the viscoelastic properties of the skin or scar. Although the Cutometer has been shown to be a reliable tool in the quantification of burn scars, there is likely a ceiling effect seen in very hard, nonpliable scars.[19,20]

The color of a scar, which is a combination of the pigmentation as well as the vascularity, may be measured with a device known as a Mexameter (Courage + Khazaka electronic GmbH, Köln, Germany). This device characterizes the color of a scar by the wavelengths of light absorbed by melanin and hemoglobin. This instrument has promising qualities for use in quantifying hypertrophic scars, but has not been shown to well discriminate between normotrophic scars and hypertrophic scars.[20] The limitations in discriminating between normotrophic and hypertrophic scars, as well as differences in opinion of the value in including color as an essential outcome for burn scars, may limit the utility of the Mexameter as a preferred measurement tool for the quantification of scar properties.[21]

The volume of a scar may be approximated by measurement of thickness through transcutaneous ultrasound. Thickness of skin or scar may be quantified by measuring the distance between the different echogenic properties of tissue within skin and scar compared with subcutaneous fat or other tissues. So far, transcutaneous ultrasound appears to be the best quantitative tool available to discriminate between normal skin, normotrophic scars, and hypertrophic scars.[20] However, because of the small area measured, a true measurement of total scar volume is not currently possible with this device.

Like the VSS, each of these instruments is limited in the degree of scarring measured. For example, the apertures of the measurement devices for the Cutometer and transcutaneous ultrasound may be 1 cm in diameter or less. As such, for scars with significant heterogeneity, such as in **Fig. 2**, a technique for repeating measurements of the same region of scar needs to be devised.

The need for clinically relevant measurement tools to describe hypertrophic scars is important outside of burns rehabilitation because hypertrophic scars may be seen in other inflammatory traumatic conditions. The hypertrophic scars seen in **Fig. 3** are the result of a complex ankle fracture and delayed wound healing. Despite the significant difference in primary injury, the scars share several characteristics with the burn scars illustrated in **Fig. 2**.

Because the viscoelastic and mechanical properties of hypertrophic scars are forever different from normal skin, extra care must be afforded to the skin in the long term. As an example, the patient in **Fig. 4** had extensive lower extremity burns 20 years and 5 months before a fall and a lower extremity fracture. The fracture was treated with open reduction and internal fixation. However, although the surgical incision healed well, in the patient's postoperative care, a tight dressing was applied over the chronic burn scar that resulted in the deep wound illustrated in **Fig. 4**.

TREATMENTS FOR HYPERTROPHIC SCAR

As noted above, a scar requires chronic maintenance and monitoring. Because sebaceous and sweat glands are not present in burn scars or burns that have been treated with autografts, the scar tends to be dry and pruritic.[22–24] As such, it is recommended that an emollient cream be applied several times per day. Furthermore, because of the skin's limited ability to participate in thermoregulation, minimization of excessive heat and sun exposure should be practiced and patients monitored for hyperthermia in extreme environments or during sport.[24,25]

The application of pressure garments has historically been a mainstay in hypertrophic scar treatment. There is some evidence that pressure may have an effect on the remodeling of hypertrophic burn scar elements such as fibrillin and elastin.[26] However, a meta-analysis of clinical studies researching the effectiveness of pressure garments suggests that overall global scar outcome measurements are not significantly different between scars treated with pressure garments and those not. In subset analysis, there may be a benefit in scar height, but very limited clinical evidence exists to support the use of pressure garments for secondary scar characteristics such as vascularity, pliability, and color. The studies included in the meta-analysis did not quantify scar characteristics, but described the outcomes using the limited clinical scales described above.[27] Clinical experience suggests that some patients find benefits other than aesthetic in wearing pressure garments, such as improvements in scar pain or itch. Others may report the pressure as significantly uncomfortable. Therefore, patients with scars may be offered pressure garments, but it is not known if they are necessary for the optimal outcome until further research is completed.

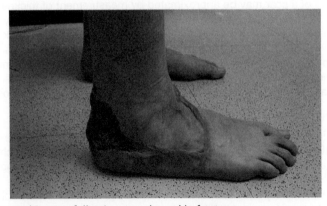

Fig. 3. Hypertrophic scars following complex ankle fracture.

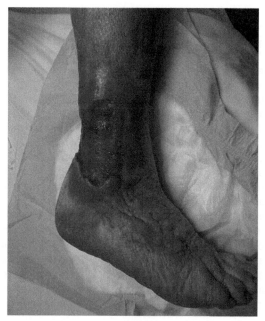

Fig. 4. New-onset deep wound in chronic burn scar.

Pruritus is a chronic problem associated with many hypertrophic scars. Beyond emollient creams mentioned above, the use of local or systemic antihistamines may be useful depending on the total body surface area involved in the areas of itchiness.[22] There is some early evidence suggesting naltrexone may be a useful treatment for burn-related itch.[28]

Corticosteroid injections and the use of pulsed dye lasers are sometimes used either alone or in combination in an effort to manage the volume and texture of hypertrophic scars. Furthermore, topical 5-fluorouracil may also be included as part of this treatment combination.[29–31] The effects of any of these treatments are unclear. Clinical deterioration with pulsed dye laser treatments has been reported.[32] Significant differences in the devices used and in the subjective nature of the outcome measures in these studies make drawing convincing conclusions difficult.

Contractures and Surgical Reconstructions

Hypertrophic scars may impair movement when they cross joints or exert abnormal forces on surrounding tissues. Contractures of the shoulder, elbow, and knee are the most common joints affected after burn injury.[33] All of the mechanisms leading to hypertrophic scar are not well understood, but contractile elements such as myofibroblasts and free actin are seen in hypertrophic scars.[34] In situ fibroblasts can have different cellular reactions depending on different culture features. For example, fibroblasts cultured in high-tension, two-dimensional environments will develop cellular features such as membrane lamella formation associated with cell migration. Fibroblasts cultured in floating, low-tension, three-dimensional matrices develop cell membrane "ruffled" morphology and fewer focal adhesions.[35]

However, it is difficult to translate the in situ burn scar fibroblast characteristics from different culture settings to the clinical application of mobilizing patients. In one in vitro model of a burn scar stretch, prolonged static stretch resulted in decreased cellular proliferation in the dermal layers, which may result in a change in the biomechanical properties of human scar.[36] Overall, there is a theoretical risk of increasing burn scar contracture by applying a mechanical stretch on a burn wound or scar, but there is a clinical risk of contracture as well as debility in immobilizing the burn patient. The ideal force, frequency, and duration of stretch to maintain joint range-of-motion while managing the cellular response to tension is not defined.

Some burn scars will impair function enough to require surgical intervention. The techniques of releasing burn scar contractures vary greatly depending on the individual characteristics of the scar in question. In general, local, linear, or small planar scars that impair movement may be lengthened by Z or V-Y plasty procedures.[37]

Historically, surgical interventions for burn scars have been postponed until the scar is considered "mature" or what may be 6 to 12 months after maturity. This was because of the concern of recurrence in the scar. This may also have been influenced by burn scar reconstructive release surgeries being performed in combination with meshed split thickness autografting.[37]

However, other surgical techniques may offer superior outcomes and offer earlier surgical reconstruction, thereby reducing the length of time of disability for the patient. For example, there are good outcomes reported with free flaps, the use of cultured or engineered skin substitutes, and tissue expansion and scar excision as part of a surgical reconstructive plan for hypertrophic scar.[38–40] There may also be a role for adjunctive pharmacotherapy such as interferon alpha in minimizing hypertrophic scar occurrence.[41]

SUMMARY

Hypertrophic scars represent an "overhealing" state in wound healing. Excessive extracellular matrix in combination with inadequate remodeling of scar tissue results in an aesthetically unsatisfactory, painful, pruritic scar that can impair function. Several treatment options are available to the rehabilitation practitioner to try to address the clinical problems posed by hypertrophic scars, but none are entirely satisfactory. An interdisciplinary clinical program, including rehabilitation physicians, surgeons, and a complementary allied health team, is necessary to address the many complications of hypertrophic scarring. Challenges to be met by the rehabilitation community include research into the quantification of burn scar measurement, the effects of mechanical forces on wound healing and scar management, and the best combination of surgical, pharmacologic, and therapy interventions to maximize outcome from burn scar reconstructive procedures.

REFERENCES

1. Bombaro KM, Engrav LH, Carrougher GJ, et al. What is the prevalence of hypertrophic scarring following burns? Burns 2003;29(4):299–302.
2. Aarabi S, Longaker MT, Gurtner GC. Hypertrophic scar formation following burns and trauma: new approaches to treatment. PLoS Med 2007;4:1464–70.
3. Miller SF, Bessey PQ, Schurr MJ, et al. National Burn Repository 2005: a ten-year review. J Burn Care Res 2006;27(4):411–36.
4. Clark RA, Ghosh K, Tonnesen MG. Tissue engineering for cutaneous wounds. J Invest Dermatol 2007;127(5):1018–29.
5. Acosta JB, del Barco DG, Vera DC, et al. The pro-inflammatory environment in recalcitrant diabetic foot wounds. Int Wound J 2008;5(4):530–9.
6. Shai A, Halevy S. Direct triggers for ulceration in patients with venous insufficiency. Int J Dermatol 2005;44(12):1006–9.

7. Verschueren JH, Post MW, de Groot S, et al. Occurrence and predictors of pressure ulcers during primary in-patient spinal cord injury rehabilitation. Spinal Cord 2011;49(1):106–10.

8. Seifert O, Mrowietz U. Keloid scarring: bench and bedside. Arch Dermatol Res 2009;301(4):259–72.

9. Engrav LH, Garner WL, Tredget EE. Hypertrophic scar, wound contraction and hyper-hypopigmentation. J Burn Care Res 2007;28(4):593–7.

10. Riordan CL, McDonough M, Davidson JM, et al. Noncontact laser Doppler imaging in burn depth analysis of the extremities. J Burn Care Res 2003;24(4): 177–86.

11. Matsumura H, Engrav LH, Gibran NS, et al. Cones of skin occur where hypertrophic scar occurs. Wound Repair Regen 2001;9(4):269–77.

12. Armour A, Scott PG, Tredget EE. Cellular and molecular pathology of HTS: basis for treatment. Wound Repair Regen 2007;15:S6–17.

13. Gabriel V. Transforming growth factor-beta and angiotensin in fibrosis and burn injuries. J Burn Care Res 2009;30(3):471–81.

14. Xie JL, Qi SH, Pan S, et al. Expression of Smad protein by normal skin fibroblasts and hypertrophic scar fibroblasts in response to transforming growth factor beta 1. Dermatol Surg 2008;34(9):1216–25.

15. Ladak A, Tredget EE. Pathophysiology and management of the burn scar. Clin Plast Surg 2009;36(4):661–74.

16. Ghaffari A, Li YY, Karami A, et al. Fibroblast extracellular matrix gene expression in response to keratinocyte-releasable stratifin. J Cell Biochem 2006;98(2): 383–93.

17. Vercelli S, Ferriero G, Sartorio F, et al. How to assess postsurgical scars: a review of outcome measures. Disabil Rehabil 2009;31(25):2055–63.

18. Baryza MJ, Baryza GA. The Vancouver Scar Scale: an administration tool and its interrater reliability. J Burn Care Rehabil 1995;16(5):535–8.

19. Nedelec B, Shankowsky HA, Tredget EE. Rating the resolving hypertrophic scar: comparison of the Vancouver Scar Scale and scar volume. J Burn Care Rehabil 2000;21(3):205–12.

20. Nedelec B, Correa JA, Rachelska G, et al. Quantitative measurement of hypertrophic scar: intrarater reliability, sensitivity, and specificity. J Burn Care Res 2008; 29(3):489–500.

21. Forbes-Duchart L, Cooper J, Nedelec B, et al. Burn therapists' opinion on the application and essential characteristics of a burn scar outcome measure. J Burn Care Res 2009;30(5):792–800.

22. Bell PL, Gabriel V. Evidence based review for the treatment of post-burn pruritus. J Burn Care Res 2009;30(1):55–61.

23. Ghahary A, Shen YJ, Wang RJ, et al. Expression and localization of insulin-like growth factor-1 in normal and post-burn hypertrophic scar tissue in human. Mol Cell Biochem 1998;183(1/2):1–9.

24. Davis SL, Shibasaki M, Low DA, et al. Sustained impairments in cutaneous vasodilation and sweating in grafted skin following long-term recovery. J Burn Care Res 2009;30(4):675–85.

25. McEntire SJ, Chinkes DL, Herndon DN, et al. Temperature responses in severely burned children during exercise in a hot environment. J Burn Care Res 2010; 31(4):624–30.

26. Costa AM, Peyrol S, Porto LC, et al. Mechanical forces induce scar remodeling. Study in non-pressure-treated versus pressure-treated hypertrophic scars. Am J Pathol 1999;155(5):1671–9.

27. Anzarut A, Olson J, Singh P, et al. The effectiveness of pressure garment therapy for the prevention of abnormal scarring after burn injury: a meta-analysis. J Plast Reconstr Aesthet Surg 2009;62:77–84.

28. Jung SI, Seo CH, Jang K, et al. Efficacy of naltrexone in the treatment of chronic refractory itching in burn patients: preliminary report of an open trial. J Burn Care Res 2009;30(2):257–60 [discussion: 61].

29. Koc E, Arca E, Surucu B, et al. An open, randomized, controlled, comparative study of the combined effect of intralesional triamcinolone acetonide and onion extract gel and intralesional triamcinolone acetonide alone in the treatment of hypertrophic scars and keloids. Dermatol Surg 2008;34(11):1507–14.

30. Darougheh A, Asilian A, Shariati F. Intralesional triamcinolone alone or in combination with 5-fluorouracil for the treatment of keloid and hypertrophic scars. Clin Exp Dermatol 2009;34(2):219–23.

31. Bloemen MC, van der Veer WM, Ulrich MM, et al. Prevention and curative management of hypertrophic scar formation. Burns 2009;35(4):463–75.

32. Allison KP, Kiernan MN, Waters RA, et al. Pulsed dye laser treatment of burn scars. Alleviation or irritation? Burns 2003;29(3):207–13.

33. Sliwa JA, Heinemann A, Semik P. Inpatient rehabilitation following burn injury: patient demographics and functional outcomes. Arch Phys Med Rehabil 2005; 86(10):1920–3.

34. Junker JP, Kratz C, Tollback A, et al. Mechanical tension stimulates the transdifferentiation of fibroblasts into myofibroblasts in human burn scars. Burns 2008; 34(7):942–6.

35. Rhee S. Fibroblasts in three dimensional matrices: cell migration and matrix remodeling. Exp Mol Med 2009;41(12):858–65.

36. Kratz C, Tollback A, Kratz G. Effects of continuous stretching on cell proliferation and collagen synthesis in human burn scars. Scand J Plast Reconstr Surg Hand Surg 2001;35(1):57–63.

37. Hudson DA, Renshaw A. An algorithm for the release of burn contractures of the extremities. Burns 2006;32(6):663–8.

38. De Lorenzi F, van der Hulst R, Boeckx W. Free flaps in burn reconstruction. Burns 2001;27(6):603–12.

39. Heimbach D, Luterman A, Burke J, et al. Artificial dermis for major burns. A multicenter randomized clinical trial. Ann Surg 1988;208(3):313–20.

40. Bozkurt A, Groger A, O'Dey D, et al. Retrospective analysis of tissue expansion in reconstructive burn surgery: evaluation of complication rates. Burns 2008;34(8): 1113–8.

41. Wang J, Jiao H, Stewart TL, et al. Improvement in postburn hypertrophic scar after treatment with IFN-alpha2b is associated with decreased fibrocytes. J Interferon Cytokine Res 2007;27(11):921–30.

FURTHER READING

Gabriel V, Holavanahalli R. Burn Rehabilitation. In: Braddom R, editor. Physical Medicine and Rehabilitation. 4th edition. Philadelphia (PA): WB Saunders.

Burn Reconstruction

Matthew B. Klein, MD, MS

KEYWORDS

• Burn • Reconstruction • Scar • Outcomes • Deformities

The tremendous advances in survival following burn injury over the past decades have shifted emphasis in care of the burn patient form survival alone to optimization of functional and psychosocial outcomes. Accordingly, reconstructive surgery plays a rightful prominent role in modern burn care. Burn reconstruction refers to the numerous procedures performed on persons with burn injuries to optimize their functional outcomes and appearance. It should be emphasized that these procedures should always be considered "reconstructive" rather than "cosmetic" because they are performed to restore what has been lost or damaged as a result of injury rather than to improve uninjured tissue for purely aesthetic reasons.

Reconstructive surgery—just as acute burn care—requires a multidisciplinary team approach. Psychological preparedness for surgery, adequate nutrition, postoperative splinting, and range of motion programs require the participation of the burn team.

TIMING OF RECONSTRUCTIVE SURGERY

Reconstructive procedures can occur several weeks to several years—even decades—following injury. There are several important considerations to selecting the appropriate time for surgery related to both the patient's physical and psychological condition. Because most burn procedures deal with issues related to scars and because the scar maturation process typically requires 12 to 18 months for completion, most procedures are not performed for at least a year following injury, as the need for procedures or the extent of procedure required may decrease over time. However, there are several important instances where surgery should be performed earlier such as in the case of exposed vital structures, severe eyelid ectropion, or unstable wounds.

There are several critical perquisites that must be met before undertaking reconstructive procedures. First and foremost is the psychological preparedness of the patient. Anatomic defects alone are not sufficient critieria to proceed with surgery. Patients need to be prepared to undergo procedures—including being prepared to return to the hospital and miss periods of work and school. Many patients will rightfully have anxiety about undergoing additional operations and have trepidation about

The author has nothing to disclose.
Division of Plastic Surgery, Harborview Medical Center, 325 9th Avenue, Box 359796, Seattle, WA 98104, USA
E-mail address: mbklein@uw.edu

Phys Med Rehabil Clin N Am 22 (2011) 311–325
doi:10.1016/j.pmr.2011.01.002
1047-9651/11/$ – see front matter © 2011 Elsevier Inc. All rights reserved.

returning to the hospital ward where they may have previously spent weeks to months. In some cases, for patients who will require many procedures over time, selecting to do a smaller procedure that does not require hospital admission and has a predictable outcome may be a reasonable first reconstruction to perform.

Patients must also have realistic expectations as to what can be achieved with each procedure. Although many patients will come to the burn reconstruction clinic with the hope that scars can be simply erased and their preinjury appearance restored, the unfortunate reality is that this will likely not be possible. Therefore, a frank discussion with the patient and his or her family is required as to what can reasonably be accomplished needs to occur. In addition, the likely need for multiple operations spread out over months to years also needs to be addressed. Often at the first visit to the burn reconstruction clinic we, along with the patient, will formulate a list of problems and potential surgeries that can be performed over time and work with the patient to prioritize these procedures. This list remains in the front of the patient chart and can be revisited and revised as needed over time. When possible, procedures should be grouped to minimize the overall number of surgeries. However, procedures that require immediate postoperative mobilization, such as joint capsulotomies and capsulectomies, should not be grouped with procedures that require prolonged postoperative immobilization like joint arthrodesis or contracture release with skin graft. There are also instances where there is no good or safe reconstructive option and this too must be carefully and thoughtfully explained to the patient. However, it is critical to still provide some hope when possible that new procedures or technologies may be developed in the future.

Special consideration needs to be made in the case of children and adolescents. It is critical that children be included in the decision-making process for surgery. Often parents will bring their children to clinic and the child may not be interested or ready for surgery. We make every effort to emphasize to parents that their child must "buy-in" to having procedures done because they are the ones having to undergo the procedure and their cooperation with postprocedural splinting and/or range of motion is also critical to the success of the procedure.

RECONSTRUCTIVE NEEDS

There are a number of common deformities that occur following burn injury that may be amenable to reconstructive surgery.

Scars and Contracture

Scarring remains the number one source of discomfort and misery for persons with burn injury (**Fig. 1**). Despite all of the advances in burn care over the past few decades and the high incidence of scarring, reported to be as high as 50% following burn injury,[1,2] there is still a limited understanding as to the risk factors and pathophysiology of scar formation. Accordingly, there exist few effective strategies to prevent scar formation and few proven strategies for treating them. Known risk factors for scarring include delay in wound closure, infection, and race (patients with pigmented skin are believed to be at higher risk for scar formation).[2,3] A number of nonsurgical therapeutic options have been described, including massage, pressure, silicone, vitamin E, and steroids. Steroid injection and topical silicone can be used on scars during the maturation process to alleviate symptoms of pain and itch and potentially reduce scar size; however, scar injection is difficult in children and may not be practical for large areas of scar. More recently, the use of lasers to improve scar appearance has been described. Parrett and Donelan[4] have reported using the pulsed dye laser to reduce scar rubor in

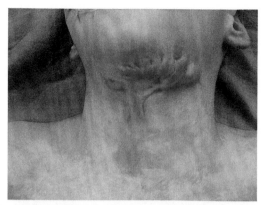

Fig. 1. Raised, red, and painful hypertrophic scar of the neck.

the early postinjury period. Whether or not treatment early on with a laser can affect ultimate scar burden remains to be seen with more experience.

Wound contraction is a natural process of shrinking that occurs in all healing tissues, whether or not they have been treated with a skin graft. Contracture refers to deformities that occur as a result of wound contraction across a joint or other mobile surface. Burn contractures occur most commonly in the hands, axilla, neck, and face. Limited contractures can often be overcome with aggressive range of motion exercises and splint immobilization; however, more extensive contractures will require surgical release. It is important to note that following surgical release, aggressive range of motion and periods of splint immobilization may be required to minimize contracture recurrence.

Pigment and Hair Loss

Problems of uneven pigment—both hyperpigmentation and hypopigmentation—are common complaints in persons with burn injury. Pigment problems can develop in areas that have healed spontaneously, areas that have undergone grafting, and in donor sites (**Fig. 2**). There are limited treatment options for pigment problems. Whitening agents such as hydroquinones have been used with some success for areas of hyperpigmentation and there have been early reports of success with dermabrading areas of hyper- or hypopigmentation and regrafting with epithelial cells obtained from the same anatomic area. However, additional clinical experience is needed to verify the success of this approach.

Hair loss can occur in areas that were burned and grafted or in areas of deep burn that healed without grafting (**Fig. 3**). Small areas of hair loss can be addressed by excision of the hairless areas and larger areas can be managed with tissue expansion, as detailed later in this article. The use of hair micrografts for eyebrows and moustache areas have also been used with success. Inappropriate hair growth in thick (ie, full-thickness) grafts can also occur. These areas can be treated with common depilatory techniques, including laser treatment or manual depilation.

Pain and Itch

Pain and itch remain common complaints even years after burn injury. Although wounds may be all closed and scars well matured, patients will still complain of persistent pain and itch. If pain and itch occur in a discrete area of scar then surgical excision

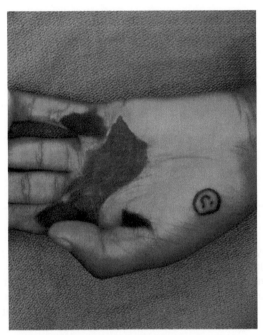

Fig. 2. Hyperpigmented full-thickness skin grafts of the palm.

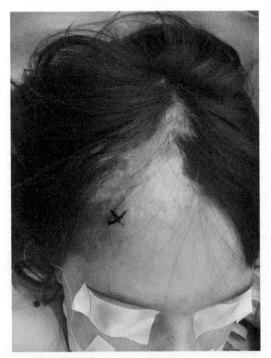

Fig. 3. Burn alopecia of the scalp of a young girl. Given the small area of hair loss, this patient was managed with excision of the area without hair.

of the scar may provide significant relief. Similarly, pain associated with a contracture deformity may also resolve with surgical correction. However, pain alone should not be an indication for surgery. In the absence of a visible deformity that can be corrected surgically, undertaking a procedure to relieve pain may prove fruitless.

OVERVIEW OF TECHNIQUES FOR RECONSTRUCTIVE SURGERY

There are a number of common techniques used in burn reconstructive surgeries. A brief description of the most common techniques used is provided in the following sections.

Scar Release and Excision

Scar contracture release is usually achieved by incising the scar band at its point of maximal tension. Given that contracture bands typically exist in a larger area of scar, releasing incisions are often extended to tissue beyond the scar band itself. Full release requires that incision be carried completely through the scar tissue until healthy tissue is reached. In some cases, release of the subcutaneous tissue and muscle fascia may also be required to achieve full release. This is often the case in the neck and axilla. Long-standing deformities of the digits may also require dividing the scar around the tendons and joint capsules and the surgeon must be aware of the potential need to divide these underlying structures and challenges in covering the subsequent defect, as skin grafting is not possible on exposed tendon, bone, and joint.

For broad areas of scar, total scar excision is necessary and practical. These procedures are relatively straightforward and have predictable results. However, although they may be relatively simple from a technical standpoint, they can provide tremendous relief to patients suffering from pain and itch from a hypertrophic scar. There are 2 general approaches to scar excision—extralesional and intralesional. Extralesional excision refers to excision of the entirety of the scar and suturing together healthy, unscarred tissue (**Fig. 4**). In contrast, intralesional excision refers to excision of most of the scar but a rim of scar is left behind and sutured together. The purported benefit of intralesional excision is that there will be no new tissue injury—incision is made through previously scarred tissue only and therefore the process of scar formation has already occurred in this tissue and is unlikely to recur. The relative risks and benefits of each approach should be discussed with the patient before surgery. Many scars are too large to be removed in one setting and often require several "serial" excisions. We typically wait 8 to 12 months between serial excisions so the tissue can sufficiently heal and soften so that it can be optimally mobilized again to achieve closure.

Wound Closure

There are a number of different approaches to achieving wound closure that vary in complexity from relatively simple to technically demanding. Reconstructive surgery requires a systematic and principle-based approach to accurately evaluate each reconstructive problem and formulate an effective treatment plan. Following is a discussion of the most common approaches to wound closure.

Skin grafts

Skin grafts remain the most common technique for coverage for burn deformities— particularly because the defect in most cases resulted from the loss of skin. Skin grafts are broadly classified as either split thickness or full thickness depending on the amount of dermis included in the graft. Skin grafts are obtained from an area referred

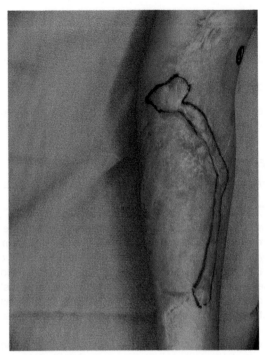

Fig. 4. Excision of a rim of hypertrophic scar of the forearm. This is an extralesional excision that includes the margins of the scar.

to as the donor site and transferred to the recipient site. For skin graft take to occur, the recipient wound bed must be well vascularized; skin grafts will not take on areas of exposed bone or tendon. In addition, the amount of contraction that occurs at the graft recipient site is inversely related to the thickness of the graft. Therefore, ideally, thick grafts are used following contracture release because the more dermis present in a graft the less contraction that occurs during the healing process. Full-thickness grafts are generally reserved for small areas (on the hand and face in particular) so that full-thickness skin graft donor site can be closed primarily. Evaluation of potential donor sites is a critical component of reconstructive surgery planning because patients who have had extensive burn injuries may have few available donor site areas. Patients should be given a choice of donor sites when multiple options exist but it is important to ration donor sites appropriately based on the need for other potential procedures. For example, we will reserve the scalp if we anticipate needing to graft large areas on the face because the scalp provides an ideal color match for the face.

Skin substitutes

Skin substitutes—particularly dermal substitutes—have long been used in the management of both acute burn wounds and burn reconstruction with the purported benefits of less donor site and recipient site scarring. Dermal substitutes are particularly useful in cases of donor site deficiency, such as when the patient has sustained an extensive injury. Given the benefits of using thicker skin grafts with more dermis to minimize contraction and recurrent contracture, dermal substitutes offer a potential advantage when thick split-thickness donor sites are not available. However, there are drawbacks to the use of skin substitutes including infection risk and usually the need for more than one surgical procedure—one for application of the material and the second for skin grafting following a period of time to allow for adequate vascularization.

Z-plasty and Y-V-plasty

Local tissue rearrangement is a common procedure done to address burn scar deformities. The 2 most useful procedures are Z-plasty and Y-V-plasty; each has its distinctive geometric properties and relative benefits. It is important to emphasize that these procedures are well suited to address scar bands because they both reorient and lengthen scars but are not appropriate options for cases of significant scar contracture that require release and the provision of additional tissue in the form of skin graft or other tissue flaps. Areas with even moderate degrees of missing tissue will be inadequately addressed by a Z-plasty and require the addition of soft tissue. The principal drawback to Z-plasty use is that transposition and advancement of the Z-limbs require extensive undermining and this often means undermining scar that can result in partial flap ischemia. For this reason, in many cases we prefer to use Y-V plasties because they require minimal flap undermining to achieve the desired advancement.

Other flaps

Other soft tissue flaps that may include skin, fascia, and muscle can be used for wound closure. These flaps can be obtained locally from areas adjacent to the contracture site or from donor sites far from the contracted area. The use of microsurgical tissue transfer may be needed in certain cases when there are no reasonable local tissue options. Fascial flaps, such as the radial forearm flap, are very useful for providing thin pliable coverage following contracture release or for lining of facial structures such as the nose. Muscle flaps are particularly useful for areas with significant contour deformity that require bulky soft tissue. Muscle flaps are also useful for breast reconstruction (as described later in this article) and to cover chronically exposed joints.

Tissue expansion

Tissue expansion is a useful technique for wound closure in areas where primary closure is difficult to achieve and there is insufficient tissue for local flaps. Tissue expansion is a technique in which healthy, uninjured tissue is gradually expanded by a silicon implant so that additional tissue can be generated that can be used to close an adjacent defect. Tissue expanders come in a variety of sizes and shapes and expander selection is based on anatomic area and amount of tissue needed. Tissue expansion is particularly useful for reconstruction of the head and neck where the use of tissue similar in color and texture can significantly enhance the surgical outcome (**Fig. 5**). Tissue expansion is also the most effective method for treating large areas of burn alopecia as explained later in the discussion of scalp reconstruction. It is important to note that tissue expansion is a time-intensive endeavor for both the surgeon and the patient. Two operations are needed—one for expander placement and one for expander removal and weekly visits are needed to gradually fill the tissue expander. Therefore, if most of a scar can be excised in 2 operations, this is likely a better option than tissue expansion.

There are several important caveats to tissue expansion. First, there must be adequate healthy tissue available to undergo expansion. Scarred wounds and grafts are not good candidates for expansion. In addition, expansion of distal extremities has been reported to be associated with significantly high rates of expander extrusion and other complications. Patients must also be prepared to come to the clinic on a weekly basis over the course of several weeks to months to undergo expansion

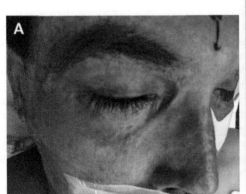
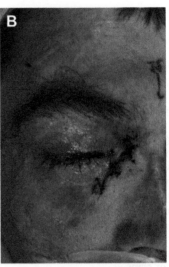

Fig. 5. A medial canthal web (*A*), which was treated by Z-plasty rearrangement (*B*).

and children must be able to be still enough to cooperate with the filling of the expanders.

POSTOPERATIVE REHABILITATION: SPLINTS AND RANGE OF MOTION

The ultimate outcome of any reconstructive endeavor requires a coordinated effort among the surgical team, the therapy team, and the patient. The success of even the most well-planned and technically executed surgical procedure is contingent on an effective postoperative plan that incorporates the principles of rehabilitation. A detailed discussion with the patient and the burn center therapists should occur preoperatively so that a plan for postoperative immobilization and subsequent mobilization can be formulated. In many instances, we will instruct patients and (in the case of children) parents on the types of exercises that will be required following surgery and have them begin to incorporate these exercises into their daily routine. This is particularly important in the case of children who may have developed contractures owing to a lack of diligent range of motion therapy. In some cases we will not perform any reconstructive procedures until it is clear that that there will be postoperative compliance with the therapy regimen. It must be clearly articulated that surgery is not a substitute for range of motion therapy. Furthermore, patients may select to delay their surgeries until a time when it is convenient to undergo a period of immobilization such as during school vacations.

Typically, following contracture release, immobilization occurs for the first 5 to 7 days postoperatively to allow for adequate healing to occur. During this period, patients are immobilized in a position that optimizes function, which may or may not be a position that optimizes comfort. For example, the axilla will be splinted in 100 or more degrees of shoulder abduction, the neck in mild hyperextension, and the eyelids will be kept on maximal stretch with traction sutures. Once graft/flap take has been achieved, mobilization occurs. Although physical and occupational therapists are of incredible value in helping patients achieve maximal function, it is critical for patients to be instructed on range of motion exercises and be encouraged to perform them multiple times a day—not just when in therapy sessions. We will typically have patients wear splints for weeks to months following contracture release to minimize contracture recurrence. Patients are instructed to remove the splints for range of motion exercises but then to replace them. It is common that splints will need to be adjusted or remade during the scar maturation process and patients are therefore encouraged to bring splints with them to each clinic visit.

COMMON RECONSTRUCTIVE PROBLEMS AND PROCEDURES

Reconstructive burn surgery—as is true for all of plastic surgery—requires a principled approach to patient evaluation and surgical plan formulation. Persons with burn injury provide special challenges in terms of the extent and complexity of scar deformities and the potential lack of healthy tissue that could be used in reconstructive procedures. In the following sections we provide a description of the most common deformities and their treatments by anatomic area.

Head and Neck

Scalp

Burn alopecia (baldness) results from deep burns of the scalp. Clearly, acute burns that are excised and grafted are incapable of hair growth and wounds that are deep and heal spontaneously may also become areas of alopecia. There are 2 main strategies for addressing burn alopecia—serial excision and tissue expansion. Serial excision refers to the excision of areas of tissue over multiple repeat (ie, serial) procedures. This approach is most effective and practical for smaller areas of alopecia that may be eliminated in one or two procedures. Larger areas of alopecia typically require tissue expansion of remaining hair-baring scalp. Significant alopecia (more than half of the scalp) may require more than one tissue expander treatment. As discussed previously, it is important to note that tissue expansion requires a significant commitment on the part of the patient and his or her family. Expansion usually occurs over the period of several weeks to months. In addition, expanders placed under areas of scar may also be subject to infection or exposure. We typically do not perform expansion in infants and toddlers because of potential difficulties children have with cooperation, both with the installation of fluid and with avoiding activity that may lead to injury to the head and expander rupture. Often for children with extensive alopecia not yet candidates for expanders, we will begin by performing serial excisions to begin to reduce the burden of alopecia.

Facial defects

Acute and reconstructive burn surgery of the face is probably the most challenging aspect of burn care. Facial burn results can be critical to appearance and to feelings of self-esteem. Furthermore, facial scar deformities may be the most difficult to correct completely.

Eyelids and Eyebrows

Eyelid deformities following facial burns occur quite frequently. Eyelid position can be affected not only by eyelid burns themselves—with loss of skin and other lid structures—but also from scarring of the cheeks and forehead. Cicatricial ectropion can result from the downward pull on the lid from a scarred cheek or the upward pull of the upper lid from a contracted forehead wound. When evaluating the patient with lid deformity, one must assess the ability of the patient to close the lids completely to adequately protect the underlying conjunctiva and globe. Inability to adequately protect the globe is one of the few indications for early reconstructive surgery. It is important to note that minimal lid deformities may indeed improve over time with massage and scar maturation.

Surgical management of ectropion requires release of the scar tethering the lid so it can be returned to its normal anatomic position and then skin grafting of the resulting soft tissue defect. Full-thickness skin grafts harvested from areas above the clavicles (ie, neck, posterior ear) typically provide the best result. We typically do not operate on both eyes at the same time because usually the eyes are covered with occlusive dressings for 5 to 7 days postoperatively and we are reluctant to completely occlude a patient's vision even for this brief period of time.

Another common lid deformity is the medial canthal web. In fact, when both the lids and nose require grafting some webbing invariably develops. We treat these webs by either Y-V plasty along the length of the web or a double-opposing Z-plasty (see **Fig. 5**). Both procedures disrupt and reorient the scar band in this area and tend to be highly effective.

A portion or the entirety of the eyebrow may be missing following a deep face burn. There have been several techniques described for addressing missing eyebrows, including the use of strip grafts of the scalp (as described by Brent[5]), island flaps from the temporal scalp, and micrografting of scalp hair follicles. When reconstructing the brow, care must be taken to ensure that the hairs are placed in the correct orientation for the eyebrow. Patients need to be advised that transplanted hair may grow and require intermittent trimming. Other patients will elect to have eyebrows permanently tattooed in lieu of surgery.

Nose and Lips

Defects of the nose can be quite challenging. The most common deformity is alar retraction—essentially a scar contracture of the alar rim. The most effective way to deal with this deformity is to recreate the ala by grafting skin and cartilage. More complex nasal deformities include a shortened tip and wide-appearing nasal dorsum. In fact, severe facial scar contracture in children can deform the nasal bones and require nasal osteotomies to reposition the bones and narrow the dorsum once young adulthood is reached. Taylor and colleagues[6] recently described a scar-revision technique using an inferior-based nasal turndown flap to address the common nasal deformities, including the widened dorsum.

Subtotal or total destruction of the nose may require total nasal reconstruction including replacement of nasal lining, cartilage support, and skin cover. Basic principles for total nasal reconstruction as described in most plastic surgery texts need to be followed; however, it is rare that the remainder of the face has sufficient healthy tissue available to use for reconstruction. In these cases, distant tissue—including microvascular free flaps—can be used to provide both lining and skin cover. One must also consider nasal prostheses either as a temporary measure until the patient is physically and psychologically prepared for a series of extensive reconstructive procedures or even as a permanent treatment.

There are several common lip deformities following burn injury including upper and lower lip ectropion, microstomia, loss of the philtral columns and dimple, and loss of the mental crease. Ectropion of the lips is generally treated by release of the scar and full-thickness skin grafts. However, in the case of lower lip ectropion, if there is also a severe neck contracture this may need to be addressed before the lip, as described later in this article.

Commissuroplasty is used to address burn microstomia. The appropriate location of the commissure is identified by drawing a line from the medial limbus down to the lip. A triangle of scar can then be removed with the apex at the point of the medial limbus and then a flap of oral mucosa is advanced outward to close the defect and recreate the commissure. The philtrum itself can be recreated by using a skin graft the shape of the philtrum or using a philtral-shaped cartilage graft. Philtral reconstruction can be performed simultaneously with the remainder of the upper lip or (more preferably) at a second operation once adequate lip length is established.

Ears

Ear deformities can vary from relatively small problems with simple solutions, such as adherence of the ear to the mastoid, to complex problems, such as severe cartilage deficiency with significant deformity. In cases of adherence of the ear to the mastoid area or lack of ear projection, the adherence can be divided and a full-thickness skin graft placed to elevate the ear and achieve optimal angle with the scalp. Cases of extensive ear deformity can be more challenging. The use of cartilage grafts to recreate the helix can be performed but typically there is a lack of adequate soft tissue coverage since the adjacent skin, including the temporoparietal region, may also be scarred. Therefore, in cases of extensive ear deformity, a prosthesis, either partial or complete, should be considered.

Other Facial Areas

Defects on the cheeks may vary from small patches of hypertrophic scar to large areas of scar that may involve the entirety of the cheek. Small areas of scar can be excised and closed as described previously (either intralesionally or extralesionally). However, larger areas of hypertrophic scar will require excision and grafting or tissue expansion of local uninjured skin. Spence[7] provides a useful approach to reconstruction of the entire face—including the cheek regions. He has had a great deal of success by using tissue expanders in the shoulder/scapula region and using this tissue to resurface large areas of the face.

Face Transplantation

There is growing interest in the potential benefit of face transplantation for persons with burn injury. The technical expertise required to harvest and successfully transplant soft tissue alone or soft tissue and bone has long existed; however, there are a number of practical considerations that need to be adequately addressed. First, there may be few patients who would actually benefit from transplantation of the entire face. Furthermore, because most burn scar deformities involve only the soft tissue, it is unclear of what the aesthetic outcome would be of transplanting soft tissue from another person onto one's bony foundation. The current status of immunosuppression regimens would require a transplant recipient to be on lifelong immunosuppressive drugs with well-known untoward side effects. Finally, if a face transplant were to fail—either for technical or physiologic reasons—the result could be devastating in terms of appearance, function, and psychological health. Therefore, whereas there is excitement about the potential benefit of face transplantation, efforts at this time should focus on development of standards for patient evaluation and selection that address patient expectations, psychological preparedness, and likelihood of complying with posttransplant immunosuppressive regimens, which are critical as the field of face transplantation evolves.

Neck

Neck contractures are one of the most common complications of burn injury. Neck contractures can be highly disfiguring and significantly affect function—both neck range of motion and oral competence. Neck reconstructive surgery has 2 distinct components: scar release and wound closure. Adequate scar release is essential to preventing recurrent contracture. Complete neck scar release requires division of the scar, which may extend through the neck skin and subcutaneous tissue to the platysma or even deeper. Once full release is achieved, selection of appropriate tissue for wound closure is needed. A number of different approaches to neck contracture management have been described, including use of grafts, skin substitutes, and free tissue transfer. Aggressive range-of-motion therapy usually begins 5 to 7 days following neck release and patients may need to wear a custom neck splint for months following surgery to minimize repeat contracture.

BREAST RECONSTRUCTION

Breast deformities can vary from the presence of small areas of hypertrophic scar to missing nipple-areola complex to complete amastia. Burned breast reconstruction can be quite challenging and require multiple procedures staged over several years. Breast development can be affected by both injury to the breast bud in young girls and to surrounding scar that may restrict breast growth. As soon as bulging on the chest occurs suggestive of breast development, scar release and grafting of the chest should be performed to try to provide adequate compliance to allow breast growth (**Fig. 6**). In cases of unilateral amastia, one should wait to perform breast reconstruction until the contralateral breast growth is complete so that symmetry can be established. Reconstruction can then be performed using implants and/or autologous tissue reconstruction. It is critical that patients understand the rationale behind the timing and staging of breast reconstruction and be aware of the potential for prosthetics during the time before the final stages of reconstruction.

PERINEUM

Perineal webs can occur from burns of the genitalia and/or perineum as well as from deep burns of the proximal medial thigh. Perineal webs interfere with hygiene and can also affect ambulation. Early scar release and skin grafting is often necessary in cases of severe deformities. Contracture of the labia and the scrotum typically occur from webbing in the inguinal region and is treated by release and skin grafting. Contractures of the penile shaft can be managed as contractures elsewhere in the body—by release

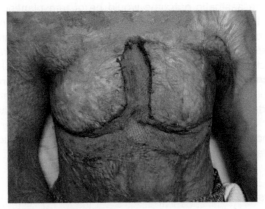

Fig. 6. Release of the developing breasts of a young woman burned as a child. This procedure separated the breast mounds and allowed for further breast development.

and skin grafting. Total phallus or scrotal reconstruction can be performed using any number of the techniques that have been described for other indications with the caveat that there may be limited suitable local tissue.

UPPER EXTREMITY

The upper extremity—and hand in particular—is commonly involved in burn injury, and scar deformities in this area can significantly impact function. Significant effort is made during the acute phases of burn management to minimize scar deformities of the hand and upper extremity; however, contractures still occur quite frequently. In fact, with survival following more extensive injuries becoming increasingly common, there is a growing complexity and number of late deformities encountered.

Axilla

Axillary contractures can occur from bands along the anterior or posterior axillary folds or—as in many cases—both. These deformities require full scar release and subsequent skin grafting or transposition of healthy tissue from the back or chest if available (**Fig. 7**). Before performing axillary release, it is very important that the patient has plateaued on range-of-motion progress. Often the more range of motion a patient has preoperatively, the better the results from surgery. In addition, the patient must be prepared to continue maximal range-of-motion exercises following release. We typically immobilize the patient for 5 days postoperatively and then begin range-of-motion therapy at that point. Splinting then continues at night for the next several months.

Elbow

Contracture of the elbow can result from scarring along the antecubital fossa and/or the dorsal aspect of the forearm and upper arm. Contracture release can be performed as described previously with the resulting defects covered with thick split-thickness skin grafts. Discrete bands may be amenable to local tissue rearrangement with Z-plasty or Y-V plasty. Heterotopic ossification (HO) of the elbow is a severe complication of burn injury and can be quite debilitating, as limited elbow range of motion can lead to limited hand use and therefore limited hand range of motion. HO results from the abnormal deposition of bone around the elbow joint and has been associated with a prolonged time to elbow wound closure.[8] A number of pharmacologic agents have been used to treat HO but with variable results. In some cases, HO will resorb on its own or with pharmacologic therapy; however, surgical correction

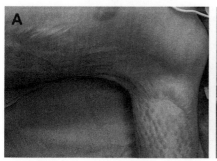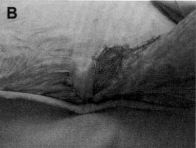

Fig. 7. Contracture of the axilla (*A*) treated by release and a combination of transposition flap of healthy skin and split-thickness skin graft (*B*).

may be necessary. Surgical correction may require extensive dissection of the elbow joint—including ulnar nerve release followed by aggressive postoperative range of motion so that intraoperative gains can be maintained.[9]

Wrist and Hand

There are a number of burn injury complications that occur in the hand and wrist that can have substantial impact on function. Areas of hypertrophic scar can be excised and closed primarily or grafted as described previously. Contractures that disrupt function can prove more challenging and often involve scarring and damage to underlying structures.

Wrist contractures occur more commonly on the wrist dorsum and are treated with release and skin grafting as described previously for other joints. However, in cases of severe contracture, scarring of the extensor tendons may also be contributing to the defect. In these cases, tenolysis is required. If the resulting defect is not able to be grafted (because of exposure of tendons or bone), then flap coverage is needed.

Flexion contractures of the digits require division—and in some cases excision—of the scar band and subsequent full-thickness skin grafts. Long-standing digital contractures may also benefit from temporary (3–4 weeks) Kirschner-wire placement to maintain the digit in adequate position following release and graft placement. If there is indeed a joint contracture, then there is likely a significant deficit in tissue that can only be addressed by the provision of additional tissue in the form of a graft. Flexion contractures of the proximal interphalangeal (PIP) joints can also result from initial injury to the extensor mechanism itself. The well-described burn claw deformity occurs when there is subsequent hyperextension of the metacarpophalangeal joint in addition to PIP flexion deformity. Surgical reconstruction of these deformities can be quite challenging, not only because of a lack of suitable dorsal skin coverage, but also the need to reconstruct the extensor tendon apparatus and the scarred joints. PIP joint arthrodesis may be the best option, as this would provide stable, durable joint positioning.

Severe contractures may also warrant amputation. This is particularly true of the fifth digit, where patients often feel the digit "gets in the way" of performing daily tasks.

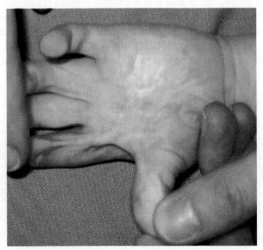

Fig. 8. Web space contracture of the thumb-index web space and contracture band along the volar aspect of the second digit.

Perhaps the most common burn reconstructive procedure performed is web space contracture release (**Fig. 8**). All 4 web spaces are prone to contracture and when this occurs there can be a significant impact on range of motion and hand function.

LOWER EXTREMITY

Lower extremity defects typically occur around the knee and foot and ankle. Scar bands in these areas are usually best treated with release and subsequent skin graft-ing. As with scar contractures along with other joint surfaces, reconstruction should be undertaken only after range of motion has plateaued, as smaller bands may be over-come with aggressive therapy. Defects of the foot and ankle similarly often require scar release and grafting with thick split-thickness skin grafts. Similar to the digits, the toe contractures are often difficult to correct, particularly if they are longstanding. To restore the toes to proper position, the extensor tendons may need to be sacrificed. If they are transected, this typically does not interfere with ambulation.

SUMMARY

The evolving shift in focus of burn care and research toward optimizing the long-term outcomes of persons with burn injuries has certainly increased the emphasis on burn reconstruction. There are an increasing number of persons surviving extensive injury who may have long-term reconstructive needs. Burn reconstruction, just as acute burn care, requires a coordinated team approach from initial consultation through recovery and rehabilitation. Clearly, in the future, one can expect evolution in surgical techniques and technologies that can improve the function and appearance of persons with burn injury.

REFERENCES

1. Spurr ED, Shakespeare PG. Incidence of hypertrophic scarring in burn-injured children. Burns 1990;16:179–81.
2. Bombaro KM, Engrav LH, Carrougher GJ, et al. What is the prevalence of hyper-trophic scarring following burns? Burns 2003;29:299–302.
3. Deitch EA, Wheelahan TM, Rose MP, et al. Hypertrophic burn scars: analysis of variables. J Trauma 1983;23:895–8.
4. Parrett BM, Donelan MB. Pulsed dye laser in burn scars: current concepts and future directions. Burns 2010;36:443–9.
5. Brent B. Reconstruction of ear, eyebrow and sideburn in the burned patient. Plast Reconstr Surg 1975;55:312–7.
6. Taylor HO, Carty M, Driscoll D, et al. Nasal reconstruction after severe facial burns using a local turndown flap. Ann Plast Surg 2009;62:175–9.
7. Spence RJ. An algorithm for total and subtotal facial reconstruction using an expanded transposition flap: a 20-year experience. Plast Reconstr Surg 2008; 121:795–805.
8. Klein MB, Logsetty S, Costa B, et al. Extended time to wound closure is associated with increased risk of heterotopic ossification of the elbow. J Burn Care Res 2007; 28:447–50.
9. Viola RW, Hanel DP. Early "simple" release of posttraumatic elbow contracture associated with heterotopic ossification. J Hand Surg 1999;24:370–80.

Psychosocial Recovery, Pain, and Itch After Burn Injuries

Shelley A. Wiechman, PhD

KEYWORDS

• Psychosocial adjustment • Burns • Pruritus • Burn pain

The average length of inpatient hospitalization for patients with burn injuries has declined during the last 10 years from 11 to 9 days.[1] This represents, on average, just more than 1 day of hospitalization per 1% burn. As a result, patients with burn injuries are being discharged with multiple, long-term, physical, and psychological challenges, such as ongoing pain, intensive physical therapy, contractures, amputations, and psychological distress. Further, issues associated with long-term adjustment have been recognized as a priority for research and clinical practice. In this article, the authors begin by using a biopsychosocial model to examine the various factors that affect burn recovery. They also discuss various aspects of pain, pruritus, sleep, and emotional distress and conclude with recommendations for treatment.

THE BIOPSYCHOSOCIAL MODEL OF RECOVERY

A person's response to stress is a function of their personality, style, and coping mechanisms and how these interact over time with the environmental factors that are present. Univariate models are insufficient to explain a person's response to a burn injury and its long-term outcomes. More sophisticated, theory-driven biopsychosocial models are needed to explain the outcomes of burn injury. Researchers have identified preburn psychological disorders, injury characteristics (eg, burn size and location, acute pain levels), lack of social support, and ineffective coping styles as risk factors for poor postinjury adjustment.

Preburn Emotional and Physical Health

A person's preburn level of physical and emotional functioning can greatly affect the course of recovery, from stay in the intensive care unit (ICU) to years after discharge. For example, patients with substance abuse disorders, diabetes, chronic obstructive

Funding support: This work was supported by the National Institute on Disability Rehabilitation Research in the Office of Special Education and Rehabilitation Services in the U.S. Department of Education.
Department of Rehabilitation Medicine, University of Washington School of Medicine, 325 Ninth Avenue, Seattle, WA 98104, USA
E-mail address: wiechman@uw.edu

Phys Med Rehabil Clin N Am 22 (2011) 327–345
doi:10.1016/j.pmr.2011.01.005

pulmonary disease, and other medical comorbidities have lower survival rates, longer lengths of stay, and fare poorer overall. The available research largely supports the impression that individuals with burns severe enough to warrant hospital care often have preexisting chaos and dysfunction in their lives. In several reviews of the literature, it was found that the incidence of mental illness and personality disorders was higher in burn unit patients than that in the general population.[2–4] For example, Patterson and colleagues[3] estimated that the presence of premorbid psychiatric disorders ranged between 28% and 75%, higher than that expected in the general population. These disorders include depression, personality disorders, and substance abuse. Another study by Patterson and colleagues[5] found that patients with burn injuries scored higher on premorbid levels of psychological distress, anxiety, depression, and loss of behavioral and emotional control than a national normative sample. These studies also found that individuals with preexisting psychopathologic conditions often cope with hospitalization through previously established, dysfunctional, and often-disruptive patterns. Such dysfunctional coping styles, in turn, had an adverse effect on the hospital course, increasing the length of stay and leading to more serious psychopathologic conditions on discharge. As an example, a burn injury and its subsequent treatment can often exacerbate anxiety in previously anxious patients. Patients with personality disorders can also struggle to cope with their burn injury and have relationship patterns with staff, which are dysfunctional and cause great difficulty for the staff. Mental health professionals need to be an integral part of the team, should help to educate burn-team members about preexisting conditions, and should understand that a person with a burn injury will not be cured of their personality disorder, mental illness, or depression, while in the burn unit.

Injury Characteristics

Researchers have begun to focus on potential variables from acute hospitalization that may have a long-term effect on adjustment.[6,7] Total burn surface area (TBSA), length of hospitalization, and days spent in the ICU or on a ventilator have been used as indicators of the severity of burn injuries. Research on the relation between these variables and outcomes has been equivocal. Patterson and colleagues[3] cautioned against using TBSA as the sole predictor of emotional outcome, citing studies that have shown significant emotional distress in persons with relatively small burns and little to no distress in persons with large burns. High inpatient pain levels have also been found to lead to long-term distress. The severity of pain that patients report in the hospital supersedes both the size of their burns and the length of hospitalization as a predictor of long-term outcome at 6 months, 1 year, and 2 years postdischarge.[6,8] Location of the burn has been found to predict adjustment, with those persons with burns on their face or hands showing more emotional distress than those with more hidden burns.[9]

Coping

In the general literature on coping, Lazarus and Folkman[10] proposed a comprehensive model of stress and coping based on the notion that a person's appraisal of the demands and consequences of a situation and the amount of control they perceive they have over the situation lead to the selection of a particular coping strategy. Several organizing terms have been used to categorize coping styles.[11] The extent to which a coping strategy involves approaching a particular stressor, rather than avoiding the stressor, is a widely used classification.[12] For instance, active strategies such as problem solving, information seeking, and social support seeking can be construed as approach-oriented coping and strategies that involve disengagement, denial, or distraction can be viewed as avoidance-oriented efforts. Neither approach-oriented nor avoidance-oriented coping behaviors are inherently adaptive or maladaptive; coping effectiveness is better determined by the characteristics of the individual and the situation.[10] However, reviews of the literature on coping with chronic illness have suggested that approach-oriented coping styles are more favorable to physical and emotional health outcomes in medical populations.[13]

Some research has suggested that the selection of a specific coping strategy depends on the individual's appraisal of the amount of control they have over the situation. For example, if a person appraises the situation as being more controllable, then they use a strategy in which they attempt to actively solve the problem or mobilize resources; if they appraise low levels of control, then they are likely to use strategies in which they distract their attention away from the stressor.[14] Little research has attempted to characterize the adaptiveness of specific coping strategies in burn patients over time. It is also unknown whether a person can be taught a specific coping style, especially when under considerable stress, such as recovering from a burn injury.

Emotional Distress

The first year or two following a burn injury appears to be a time of substantial distress.[3,15–18] Clearly, mood disorders[9,15,19–23] and anxiety disorders[15,19,20,22,24,25] are the most common symptoms of distress; however, patients may also experience myriad other problems, including sleep disturbance,[26–28] body image concerns,[29] and sexual problems.[30,31] All of these symptoms potentially contribute to decreased quality of life.[32,33]

Posttraumatic Stress Disorder

The reported frequency of acute stress disorder (ASD) following a burn injury ranges from 11% to 32%.[20,34–39] The frequency of posttraumatic stress disorder (PTSD) 3 to 6 months after a burn injury is approximately 23% to 33%,[34,40] whereas the same ranges from 15% to 45% 1 year after a burn injury.[15,20,37,41] In contrast, community-based studies show that the lifetime prevalence of persons with PTSD is 1% to 14%.[42] The large variability in reported rates of diagnosed ASD/PTSD is likely to have been caused by differences in measurement strategies and measurement time points. However, most researchers and clinicians agree that even if patients do not meet a formal diagnosis of ASD or PTSD, most burn patients have at least some of the symptoms of this disorder (eg, nightmares, intrusive thoughts, hypervigilance, avoidance) that negatively affect their quality of life. Preexisting anxiety or depressive disorders are associated with an increased risk of developing PTSD. Further, the baseline symptoms of ASD and at 1 month after discharge predict the presence of PTSD at 1 year,[43] suggesting that symptoms do not decrease over time if left untreated. In addition, burn patients with a comorbid diagnosis of PTSD are frequent users of medical services. Injury-related characteristics in burn patients, such as TBSA and the location of the injury, have repeatedly failed to predict such trauma. In contrast, issues such as the patient's mental health history, social support, and coping style hold promise as predictive factors. The authors recommend a screening tool, such as the Post-Traumatic Stress Disorder Symptom Checklist–Civilian Version (PCL-C),[44] to identify patients with symptoms of PTSD.

Depression

Research that has attempted to identify rates of depressive disorders following burn injury has been fraught with challenges. In their comprehensive review, Thombs and colleagues[45] found that most studies are from single centers, with small sample sizes and poor rates of recruitment and retention. In addition, the multiple approaches and measures used have led to a wide variation in reported rates of depressive symptoms and diagnosable disorders. For example, the range of reported symptoms in the first year after a burn injury is from 2% to 22%, and the prevalence rate after 1 year is 3% to 54%.[46] The prevalence rates of depression are much lower when a structured interview rather than a standardized measure is used. But even when standardized measures are used, the rates vary widely. The most common standardized measures are the Hospital Anxiety and Depression Scale (HADS)—depression subscale[47] and the Beck Depression Inventory (BDI).[48] The HADS does not include questions about somatic symptoms but the BDI does. It is often difficult to differentiate between the symptoms that can be attributed to the medical disorder and the somatic symptoms of depression, which could account for the higher reported rates of depression, when using the BDI rather than the HADS. Whether a measure of depression that is specific to those with burn injuries needs to be designed and validated is still under debate. The 9-item Patient Health Questionnaire is a widely used screening tool in primary care and other medical specialty clinics and may prove to be useful in the burn setting.

Several studies have also found that depression rates tend to be stable from discharge to at least the first year following a burn injury.[21] Although it is commonly assumed that these rates decrease after the first year, no longitudinal studies have reported depression rates more than 1 year postinjury. Thombs and colleagues[46] found 7 studies that reported on risk factors for depression following burn injury. As mentioned earlier, many of the identified risk factors encompass premorbid functioning, such as employment status, medical illness, and prior depression. Patients with depressive symptoms in the year before the burn injury were 5 times more likely to be diagnosed with a mood disorder at hospital discharge.[15] Other risk factors include the female gender and visible burns.[9] Although research in this area has been fraught with methodological problems that make it difficult to pin down actual rates of depressive disorders, the authors recommend a brief screen for depressive symptoms during inpatient hospitalization, discharge, and follow-up clinic visits. Referrals to mental health professionals can be made for more in-depth assessments, if warranted by the responses on the screening tool.

Pain

It is important to discuss pain when reviewing the outcomes of burn injuries. Perry and Heidrich[49] reported that burn patients typically report their acute pain as being severe or excruciating, despite receiving opioid analgesics. However, it is important to realize that burn pain varies greatly from patient to patient, shows substantial fluctuation over time, and can be unpredictable because of the complex interaction of physiologic, psychosocial, and premorbid behavior issues.[50] Burn pain that is reported after the initial injury is not reliably correlated with the size or depth of a burn. A patient with a superficial (second degree) burn may show substantially more pain than one with a full-thickness (third degree) burn, because of both physical (eg, location and mechanism of the injury, individual differences in pain threshold and tolerance, response to analgesics) and psychological factors (eg, previous pain experiences, anxiety, depression). Indirect assessments of pain using measures of sympathetic nervous system activation (eg, hypertension, tachycardia, tachypnea) that may be of value in other acute pain settings are notoriously inaccurate in the patient with burn injuries because of the complex metabolic response. As a result, it is critical to realize that predicting the amount of pain or suffering that a patient will experience based on the nature of or the physiologic response to the burn injury is not possible, and furthermore, the patient's pain experience can change dramatically during the course of both inpatient and outpatient care. It is also important to note that pain can continue well after wound healing.

Because of this unpredictability, a more useful paradigm for describing acute burn pain is based on the clinical settings in which it commonly occurs. This approach is also useful because analgesic treatment decisions can also be based on such a classification. Thus, burn pain is generally classified into 5 clinical settings[51]:

1. Background: pain that is present while the patient is at rest, results from the thermal tissue injury itself, and is typically of low-moderate intensity and long duration (until the burn wound is healed)
2. Procedural: a brief but intense pain generated by wound care (eg, debridement, dressing change) or rehabilitation activities (physical and occupational therapies)
3. Breakthrough: an unexpected spiking of pain levels that occurs when analgesic efforts are exceeded, either at rest or during procedures
4. Postoperative: a predictable and temporary (2–5 days) increase in pain complaints following burn excision and grafting, in large part because of the creation of new wounds in the processes of skin graft harvesting and autografting
5. Chronic: pain that lasts longer than 6 months or remains after all burn wounds and skin graft donor sites have healed, and is thus a challenge primarily in the outpatient setting.

Chronic burn pain warrants further discussion because it has the greatest effect on the rehabilitation phase of recovery. The mechanisms and treatment of chronic burn pain are inadequately studied and poorly understood. Although most acute burn pain results from tissue damage, it is important to be aware that pain from nerve damage may also be present, particularly in severe injuries associated with extremity amputations, and represent an anatomic source for chronic burn pain complaints. Because there are identifiable sensory changes in patients with burn injuries, it is unclear whether these patients' pain should be defined as chronic pain or simply as an ongoing form of acute or neuropathic pain. Regardless of the label used to classify postburn injury chronic pain, ongoing pain has the potential to have a significant negative effect on the quality of life of burn patients.

Malenfant and colleagues[52] found evidence for changes in the central nervous system that could maintain pain for years after a burn wound has healed. They found that significant sensory losses and sensory changes were found not only in burn sites but also in noninjured areas. Tactile sensibility deficits were significantly associated with the presence of painful sensations. This was greatest in deep burn injuries that required skin grafting.

Choiniere and colleagues[53] interviewed 104 burn patients who were in their first to seventh year post–burn injury. The mean time since burn injury was 37 months, and the mean TBSA was 19%. Surprisingly, 35% reported ongoing pain. Of those reporting pain, 75% reported interference interfered with work, 56% with sleep, and 67% with social functioning. In a sample of 236 burn patients 1 to 9 years post–burn injury with a mean time since injury of 47 months and a mean TBSA of 20%, Malenfant and colleagues[52] found a similar rate of patients with ongoing pain (36%). Work interference was reported by 67% of those with pain, 36% reported sleep difficulties, and 47% reported disturbance in social activities. Schneider and colleagues[54] reviewed the natural history of neuropathy-like pain after a burn injury. Over a 2-year period, they found 72 patients in their outpatient clinic who described symptoms consistent with neuropathic pain. The average pain rating was 7 of 10, and the pain persisted for more than 1 year after the injury. In this study, gabapentin and steroid injections were used to treat the pain in about one-third of the cases. Other interventions included rest, massage, use of pressure garments, and elevation.

Finally, Dauber and colleagues[55,56] mailed a questionnaire to members of a burn survivor support group, and of the 358 respondents, 52% reported ongoing pain, 66% said that it interfered with their rehabilitation, and 55% said the pain interfered with their daily lives. Respondents in this study also reported that thoughts of the accident and depression made their pain worse. In these studies, TBSA and skin grafting were the only predictors of chronic pain. Most respondents had not tried relaxation, imagery, or hypnosis. It is important to note that the average length of time since the burn injury in 2 of these studies was 3 to 4 years. This period is well past the 1-year time frame that medical professionals think it takes for burn injuries to be completely healed.

To provide comprehensive and consistent analgesic care for burn patients, many burn centers advocate a structured approach to burn analgesia that incorporates both pharmacologic and nonpharmacologic therapies and targets the specific clinical pain settings unique to the burn patient and yet can be individualized to meet specific patient needs and institutional capabilities. Such structured protocols help to avoid the undertreatment of burn pain that has been observed[48] when burn unit staff members fail to medicate patients adequately, despite education regarding the low risk for addictive and other side effects. There is currently no evidence to support that opioid addiction occurs more commonly in burn patients without premorbid substance abuse issues than in other patient populations requiring such analgesics for acute pain.[55] In fact, poorly treated pain in the acute setting can have long-term adverse effects. Further, neuropathic pain that goes untreated in the outpatient setting can inhibit recovery, particularly if high pain levels impair sleep and inhibit a patient's ability to participate in therapies or return to work. A discussion of specific pharmacologic treatments and protocols used to treat burn pain is beyond the scope of this article and can be found elsewhere.[57–59]

NONPHARMACOLOGIC PAIN MANAGEMENT

Before focusing on the various nonpharmacologic techniques, it is useful to understand the psychological factors that can exacerbate pain. Perhaps the most important example of such processes is the loss of control that burn patients experience and its effect on coping. Sustaining a burn injury, as well as enduring the many subsequent treatments, taxes a person's coping resources by reducing their sense of control. Most patients describe feelings of being out of control in the hospital setting because of several factors, including high pain levels, the unfamiliar environment, the dependency that patients have on their caregivers, lack of input regarding daily schedules and routines, and uncertainty about the future (eg, appearance, wound status, work, or even survival). The movement to the rehabilitation stage of recovery, whether in an inpatient unit or as an outpatient, can serve as an important step for patients, toward regaining control of their lives by promoting independence. The transition from pharmacologic treatments to the reliance on primarily nonpharmacologic treatments for pain is also an important part of this process. Many of the nonpharmacologic treatments that are used in the acute setting can continue to be useful in the rehabilitation phase.

Many choices are available when considering nonpharmacologic treatment. In choosing the most effective approach, the team should be guided by the manner in which patients typically respond to stressful medical procedures. Patient responses in these circumstances lie on a continuum ranging from giving up control to the health care professional and desiring little information to seeking out as much information as possible and participating in the procedures. Those patients who wish to give up control to the health care professional have a tendency toward cognitive avoidance and are likely to use various types of distraction techniques to avoid painful stimuli. They are said to have more of an "avoidant" coping style. Those who seek out information about the procedure and like to participate as much as they can often find distraction techniques distressing; for them, trying to ignore a procedure may amount to relinquishing too much control. Such patients are thought to have more of an "approach" coping style.[57] It is important to note that both coping styles can be adaptive and it is best for the care team to support an individual's coping style rather than try to change his/her natural response. The following paragraphs briefly describe some nonpharmacologic pain control strategies that can be helpful in the rehabilitation phase of recovery, whether it is a painful physical therapy session or an ongoing wound care.

Distraction

Various forms of distraction techniques are available. Common distraction techniques used with children include bubble blowing, singing songs, reading a story, and counting. Adults may require a bit more creativity but can engage in an enjoyable conversation, listen to music, play a video game, or immerse themselves in interactive virtual reality (VR; see later discussion) during the procedure.

Virtual Reality

Immersive VR is a technology that isolates patients from the outside world, including any threatening stimuli associated with health care. Immersive VR uses a helmet that blocks the user's view of the real world and gives the patient the illusion of going into the 3-dimensional computer-generated environment, a condition known as "presence."[60] This quality makes immersive VR particularly effective in capturing participants' attention.[60] In the burn-pain setting, the authors used a virtual environment called SnowWorld,[61] where patients float through an icy canyon and are able to direct snowballs at virtual snowmen and igloos as they appear. The image of snow was specifically chosen because its connotation of cooling is in direct contrast to the hot sensations often associated with burn pain.

The theory behind the effectiveness of VR is that attention involves the limited selection of relevant information from a variety of inputs or tasks, and each human has a finite amount of attention available.[62,63] The strength of the illusion, or presence, is thought to reflect the amount of attention drawn into the virtual world.[64] Because VR is designed to be a highly attention-grabbing experience, it reduces the amount of conscious attention available to process pain. Less attention to pain not only results in a reduction in perceived pain intensity and unpleasantness but also reduces the time patients spend thinking about their pain. VR has been shown to be effective in reducing pain in several clinical studies using it for pain distraction.[61,65–67] VR technology can also be used to administer hypnotic analgesia and is particularly effective with patients who have difficulty imagining a scene.[60]

Imagery

Imagery is simply creating or recreating an image in one's mind, presumably one that patients find pleasant and engaging. Types of imagery can be infinite and depend on the desired goals. For example, many people use healing imagery to promote this result when overcoming disease or injury. They might imagine processes, such as increased blood flow to the injured area to carry away damaged tissue and rebuild new tissue or decrease inflammation in the injured area. Although healing imagery can be an effective means of helping the burn patient feel more in control of their situation, it forces a person to focus on the injury and is therefore not a distraction technique when used in this way. In contrast, relaxation imagery tends to work best for pain control and is another form of distraction. Before a painful procedure, the clinician often talks to patients about safe or favorite places to which they can go. It can be a place where they have been before (eg, a favorite vacation spot) or simply a place that they imagine to be relaxing and safe. The clinician then collects as many details as possible about the place, such as the colors, the sounds, the smells, and objects in a place, and makes the patients practice the imagery; before the procedure, patients are encouraged to relax through deep breathing, closing their eyes, and imagining their favorite places. The patients are simply cued with the details that they have provided before beginning relaxation. Next, the patients are encouraged to imagine the place during their subsequent therapy. Children often enjoy more active forms of imagery that relate to fantasy, such as a magic carpet ride. There are also numerous imagery scripts that have been published and can be used when a person is unable to think of a safe or favorite place. These scripts usually entail a person flying or floating on a cloud through beautiful places. It is important to note that a patient should be asked about any fears, such as fear of heights, flying, or water, so that use of these images does not actually create more anxiety.

Hypnotic Analgesia

Although hypnosis involves much more than just avoidance or distraction, the end result is often similar in that this technique takes a person's focus off the painful procedure they are undergoing. Hypnosis is an altered state of consciousness characterized by an increased receptivity to suggestion, the ability to alter perceptions and sensations, and an increased capacity for dissociation. It is believed that the dramatic shift in consciousness that occurs with hypnosis is the cornerstone of an individual's ability to change the awareness of pain.[68] Hypnosis involves several stages, including building clinician-patient rapport, enhancing relaxation through deep breathing, deepening the hypnotic state and narrowing the patient's attention, providing posthypnotic suggestions, and alerting.[69] Posthypnotic suggestions permit hypnosis at any time before a painful procedure, thus eliminating the need for the clinician's presence during the procedure. The authors use a rapid induction analgesia format described by Patterson[69] and originally published by Barber,[70] but there are numerous scripts for hypnotic analgesia that can be used directly or with improvisation. However, the technique should only be used by trained clinicians who can assess the risks and benefits of this powerful technique.

Deep Breathing

Deep breathing, also known as diaphragmatic breathing, is one of the least time-consuming techniques and the easiest technique for adults and children to learn. When a person becomes anxious and/or experiences pain, breathing becomes shallow and irregular because of the increased muscle tension in the chest wall. This type of shallow breathing, known as thoracic breathing,[71] leads to an increase in muscle tension and subsequent heightened pain. Teaching patients to have an awareness of this cycle and some deep breathing techniques that allow them to break it lead to a relaxation response that can alleviate some pain. Bubble blowing and blowing on a pinwheel are helpful tools to use with children to encourage deep breathing. Adults can be taught to place a hand on the stomach and to take a deep enough breath so that it passes through the chest and fills the stomach. The hand should rise and fall with the stomach. The exhalation is the most important part of deep breathing and should not be rushed. Diaphragmatic breathing is central to all forms of relaxation and is simple and time efficient.[71]

Progressive Muscle Relaxation

When patients are experiencing stress, such as pain, they tend to use muscles inefficiently,[71] resulting in muscle bracing that can lead to an increase in pain. Progressive muscle relaxation is a technique developed by a physician, Edmund Jacobson,[72] after observing increased muscle tension in hospitalized patients and discovering that more-tense patients took longer to recuperate and had poorer outcomes. He taught patients to systematically focus on a muscle group, tense and relax it, and then progress to a different group. This progression usually starts with the distal muscle groups and moves to the proximal ones until total body relaxation is achieved. Most patients are able to learn this technique with practice, using a prewritten or individually tailored script or independently using commercial audiotapes. If a person is unable to actively tense a muscle group because of pain or injury, he/she can still imagine each muscle becoming progressively warm, heavy, and relaxed, a process known as autogenic training. The patients repeat each statement to themselves as they hear it in on a tape (eg, "My right hand is heavy, my right hand is relaxed, my right hand is becoming warm…").

Quota System

The quota system is an operant technique often used by burn care providers to promote a sense of mastery among patients undergoing painful wound care procedures and difficult physical therapies.[73] Caregivers are encouraged to pace their procedural demands in a manner that is consistent with the individual's level of tolerance by taking baseline measurements for each task that needs to be performed and gradually (10% per day) increasing the demands of each task. Rest is used as the reinforcement for successfully reaching a quota or in other words, meeting a predetermined task. Goals for each task are determined based on what was done the previous day, and patients are expected to work until the goal is accomplished rather than work until they feel pain or fatigue. This technique puts more control in the hands of the patient, preventing a syndrome of learned helplessness that can often develop because of painful therapies. It also avoids reinforcing pain behaviors. The quota system is based on the notion that although physical therapies after a burn injury are painful, this pain itself is not damaging and does not negatively affect outcome.

Positive Reinforcement

Another operating principle that is often successful with patients with burn injuries, particularly children, is positive reinforcement. There is no intrinsically rewarding aspect of a burn injury or burn recovery. In fact, children often see the treatment for a burn injury as a punishment. Therefore, children need to be rewarded for participation in the recovery process and for displaying appropriate behavior. For example, it is common in a rehabilitation unit to find a sticker board and prize box in each child's room. Behavioral expectations are established in advance and define the responsibilities the child has for that day, including wound care, physical and occupational therapy, eating meals, and so forth. They receive rewards (stickers) for each responsibility that is accomplished. Once they have a set number of stickers, they are able to pick a bigger prize from the prize box, which is known as establishing a token economy. Other creative means of positive reinforcement can also be effective, such as reading stories, watching movies or television, or offering adult attention through playing a game or reading a story. When children are frequently reinforced for good behavior or after completing a therapeutic goal, it lessens the need for punishment for bad behavior and makes the therapy more tolerable.

Cognitive Restructuring

Cognitive restructuring is frequently used as a coping technique for patients with chronic pain.[74,75] There are reports in the literature of the use of this technique for coping with various type of pain, including pain from dental and surgical procedures.[76] A handful of studies have analyzed this approach for burn pain.[77,78] Catastrophizing has been found to have the strongest link between thoughts and pain. This distorted thinking style exaggerates any sensation of pain or a setback and becomes a point of perseveration for the patient. For example, a minor setback in therapy following a planned surgery (such as a contracture release), a wound infection, or simple fatigue can turn into thoughts such as "I can't take this anymore; I have to start all over again; I will never recover."

The first step in cognitive restructuring is to identify and stop negative catastrophizing thoughts, such as "this is really going to hurt" and "I can't handle this pain," that only lead to an increase in anxiety and a subsequent increase in pain. Patients can learn to recognize these negative thoughts and stop them, perhaps by picturing a stop sign or red light in their mind. They can also distract themselves by turning their attention to another topic. Children as young as 7 years have been taught to use this technique successfully.[77,79]

Ideally, the authors want patients to transform their catastrophic thoughts into positive statements. This is known as reappraisal or reframing. For example, they may change the negative thought in the previous example to "I have been through this wound care procedure before and it did not hurt as much as I thought it would" or "I have a very high pain tolerance and can cope with whatever will happen." Patients may also benefit from being taught the difference between hurt and harm, when interpreting their pain sensations.[80] Specifically, an increase in pain is often a good sign with respect to burn wound healing. As discussed earlier, deep (third degree) burns often destroy nerve endings and limit the capacity for nociception. In deep burns that begin to heal or in more shallow burns, skin buds develop, which are highly innervated and sensitive to pain and temperature.[69] Explaining this healing process to patients can help them to understand the nature of their pain and to reframe negative thoughts into reassuring positive ones.

Participation

Allowing patients who have more of an approach coping style to participate in their own burn care and recovery is one of the simplest and most effective ways to increase their sense of control and reduce anxiety. The authors often use the technique of "forced choice" for children to create more of a sense of control over their environment, without overwhelming them with choices. When a child needs to accomplish an unpleasant task, parents and caregivers can create a situation whereby the child is given 2 choices in how to proceed with the task. For example, a child who is having difficulty in physical therapy may be given the choice of having the therapy before lunch or after lunch, or picking the exercise that they start with. This method is likely to fail if more than 2 choices are given or if a child is presented with an option that caregivers or parents have no intention of allowing. Setting rehabilitation goals is also an area where patients, particularly adults, should be allowed to participate. Patients will be more motivated to work to achieve the rehabilitation goals if they have helped to define them. Goals are very individual, and each patient will have different goals depending on their priorities and their level of desired independence. For example, a mother of young children may have a goal of regaining enough strength and function to lift her baby, whereas a construction worker may have a goal of being able to grip a hammer or other tools.

Recently, there have been several rigorous systematic reviews of studies that have focused on both pediatric and adult nonpharmacologic pain management strategies. Hanson and colleagues[81] conducted a systematic review of nonpharmacologic interventions for acute procedural pain in pediatric patients with burn injuries. Using the systematic review methods of the US Preventive Services Task Force, they found 12 articles that met the study criteria, and 7 of the 12 articles were rated as fair or good. They categorized these 12 articles into child-mediated, parent-mediated, and health care provider–mediated interventions. Of the child-mediated interventions, both VR distraction and stress management showed promising results. Of the health care provider interventions, massage therapy and optimizing patient control during wound care were effective in relieving wound care pain when compared with a control group. Parent-mediated interventions were not found to be effective, and in fact, one study showed an increase in distress in children when parents were present.[82] Although the study designs in these interventions were rated as poor, the findings are consistent with those reported by clinicians, in that parental presence during painful procedures can either help a child or hurt a child, depending on the parents' affect and ability to soothe their child. This is a difficult intervention to study but one that deserves more attention in this era of family-centered care and emphasis on increased parental involvement in a child's care. It would be a tremendous benefit to the field if the variables that are necessary to facilitate a positive parental presence and the variables that serve as barriers to the success of this treatment could be determined. Hanson and colleagues[81] acknowledged that it was very difficult to conduct randomized controlled trials with adequate sample sizes in this population, but there is need to find empirical support for the techniques that are chosen.

de Jong and colleagues[83] also conducted a systematic review of the literature for nonpharmacologic interventions for acute burn pain in adults. They found that hypnosis was the most frequently studied intervention and that most studies on hypnosis showed a beneficial effect when compared with a control group. They concluded that hypnosis seems to have a strong effect on the affective component of pain. Their review also showed beneficial effects through distraction relaxation and found that any technique that enhances a patient's control over the situation is beneficial.

The investigators of these systematic reviews have provided directions for future research that would advance knowledge of the effectiveness of nonpharmacologic interventions. These suggestions included the need for large sample sizes, documentation regarding study response rates and randomization methods, experimental control for premorbid psychosocial variables, details on instructions given to patients, cost outcomes, and assurance of treatment integrity/adherence.[81,83]

SLEEP

Sleep problems are one of the most common complaints of burn patients once they are discharged from the hospital, yet probably one of the most undertreated. Sleep problems are best viewed as a symptom rather than a disease and are frequent even in the absence of burn injury, affecting up to 50% of normal adults in the United States.[84] Sleep problems in a general population, such as insomnia, can lead to distress, impaired functioning, increased accidents, and decreased work productivity.[85,86]

With burn patients, poor sleep can affect issues, such as therapy performance, pain control, adjustment, and even wound healing. Thus, addressing sleep problems after burn injuries is an important issue, in addition to the variety of other complications that patients have to face.

A burn injury and its treatment present a multitude of factors that can interfere with sleep. Early in treatment, the hospital setting and the nature of care can be highly disruptive factors. Frequent painful and intrusive treatments, noisy settings, metabolic imbalance, and awakening to take vital signs are the rule rather than the exception. As wounds heal, pruritus (itch) can become extremely unpleasant, in addition to the pain. Anxiety and depression can by themselves interrupt sleep, but medications to control burn-related complications, such as pruritus, pain, and depression, also have an effect on sleep. Thus, patients with burn injuries experience impaired sleep for long periods, first from the issues associated with hospitalization and later as a function of the transition to home.

Given all these factors, it is not surprising that the few studies that have been done on sleep quality of burn patients reflect high levels of disruption. Rose and colleagues[87] followed up 82 children with severe burn injuries and reported serious sleep disturbances 1 year after injury. The sleep disturbances included nightmares, bed-wetting, and sleepwalking. Approximately 63% of the patients complained of needing daytime naps, which is far greater than the norm.[88] The few studies that have monitored polysomnography in burn patients have reported increased total sleep time, decreased stages 3 and 4 sleep, decreased rapid eye movement sleep, and increased arousals when compared with age-matched controls.[89–91]

In treatment of sleep disorders after burn injuries, there is little question that health care professionals entertain pharmacologic options far too early and to the exclusion of more benign options. Clinicians should work with the patients on nonpharmacologic interventions before choosing this option. Nonpharmacologic options include sleep hygiene, stimulus control, sleep restriction, relaxation therapy, cognitive-behavioral therapy, and light therapy. Sleep hygiene interventions include changing the environment (eg, quiet rooms), reducing daytime naps, establishing regular sleep-wake schedules, reducing stimulant consumption from late afternoon to before bedtime when appropriate (eg, caffeine, candy, nicotine, alcohol), decreasing stimuli at night (eg, Internet, television), and proper timing of food and exercise. Stimulus control involves creating the bed as a stimulus for sleep by having the patient go to bed only when sleepy and removing competing stimuli from the bedroom (eg, television); sleep restriction focuses on having the patient remain in bed only when asleep. Cognitive-behavioral therapy can help patients work with the dysfunctional thoughts that disrupt sleep, relaxation therapy is self-explanatory, and light therapy can address disruption of circadian rhythms. A full review of the medications used to treat sleep disorders after burn injury is reported by Jaffe and Patterson.[28]

PRURITUS

Pruritus continues to be one of the most common and distressing complications following burn injury. Pruritus can be severe. It interferes with sleep and daily activities and can reopen wounds because of scratching. Postburn pruritus also tends to be cyclical, in that it begins in the early stages of wound healing, peaks at 6 months postburn, and declines after the first year following the injury.[92] Pruritus occurs in both healed and grafted skin but is more intense where hypertrophic scarring has formed. There is a paucity of evidence-based research in this area, although a plethora of pharmacologic and nonpharmacologic interventions have been proposed in small-scale studies. Recently, there has been a greater understanding of the physiologic mechanisms underlying pruritus in burn injuries. For example, it is largely thought that pruritus from burns stems from inflammation, dryness, and damage to the skin, as well as nerve damage/regeneration.[93] Two review articles on evidence-based treatments for postburn pruritus have been published.[93,94] Both reviews have found some potentially promising treatments for postburn pruritus as summarized in **Box 1**. Bell and Gabriel[94] used the Practice Guidelines for burn care, 2006,[95] to classify the studies. They found the most promising treatments with the strongest study designs to be selective antihistamine receptor agonists (cetirizine/cimetidine) and pulsed dye laser. Across studies, any antihistamine administration seemed to be better than no administration, but no single antihistamine worked effectively always. Pulsed dye laser treatments were used for intense itching in smaller areas, with 3 treatments at 1-month intervals; the effects lasted up to 12 months.[96] Combinations of the various treatments may also be more effective than a single treatment from one modality.[97] The investigators caution that the evidence is based on small-scale studies, and larger, prospective, randomized controlled trials need to be conducted (see **Box 1**).

BODY IMAGE DISSATISFACTION

Burn patients frequently list the change in appearance as a major concern and source of distress. Burn injuries can cause significant changes in appearance through scarring, contractures, changes in skin pigmentation, or amputations. The effect that these physical changes have on self-esteem and body image has only recently been

---

Box 1
Treatments for pruritus under investigation

Nonpharmacologic techniques

    Laser treatment (pulsed dye)

    Transcutaneous electrical nerve stimulation

    Unna boot

    Silicone gel patch

    Massage therapy

    Pressure garments

    Hypnosis

Topical treatments

    Doxepin cream

    Local anesthetics (lidocaine/prilocaine [EMLA])

    Colloidal oatmeal

    Dapsone

    Nanocrystalline silver

    Capsaicin

Oral medications

    Ondansetron

    Antihistamines

    Gabapentin

studied.[98] Several studies of risk factors for the development of poor body image found that burn characteristics, such as the visibility of the scar, depression, female gender, and coping style, best predicted body image dissatisfaction.[99,100] An additional predictor of body image dissatisfaction is the importance that patients placed on their appearance before the burn injury. If patients had not placed much importance on their appearance before the burn injury, they tended to be much less distressed by the consequences of disfigurement.[98]

A variety of approaches have been used to address cosmetic concerns in patients in the treatment setting.[101] However, there have been no published studies on the efficacy of various treatments. Most treatments focus on cognitive-behavioral strategies to address the appraisal of a person's appearance, to teach adaptive coping strategies, and to introduce social skills that enhance self-esteem and improve social competence. The 2 programs that were designed to enhance self-esteem are the Changing Faces program in Great Britain[102] and the BEST program in the United States.[103] Both of these programs include a hospital-based image enhancement and social skills program, along with a series of publications for patients dealing with aspects of disfigurement. These programs allow people to explore their internal reactions to the responses of others toward their disfigurement and also to access several adaptive behaviors in response to the inevitable negative societal responses to disfigurement.

SUMMARY

A biopsychosocial model of burn outcomes can be useful to guide the understanding of the long-term outcomes of burn patients. The ongoing rehabilitation issues that burn patients face are complex and include physical, emotional, social, and vocational challenges. The distress of the injury does not end when patients leave the hospital. Problems with anxiety, depression, sleep, pruritus, and body image can continue for years. All these problems can affect the patient's ability to return to an acceptable quality of life. The multidisciplinary team approach to care that has long been practiced by inpatient rehabilitation units and inpatient burn units should continue after discharge. Patients can continue to benefit from the expertise provided by both burn surgeons and psychiatrists, as well as from the services of vocational counselors, social workers, physical and occupational therapists, and psychologists. Ancillary services, including support groups and peer counseling visitation, may also be useful if carefully monitored by trained professionals.[104] Finally, more research needs to focus on effective treatments for these issues. Treatment interventions for the multiple barriers that burn patients face must be sophisticated and flexible enough to account for the large variability in causes of distress.

REFERENCES

1. American Burn Association. National Burn Repository: report of data from 2000–2009. 2010. Available at: http://www.ameriburn.org/2009NBRAnnualReport.pdf?PHPSESSID=c2099c30cd05c31bd5b13650c95b4677. Accessed January 31, 2011.
2. Kolman PB. The incidence of psychopathology in burned adult patients: a critical review. J Burn Care Rehabil 1983;4:430–6.
3. Patterson DR, Everett JJ, Bombardier CH, et al. Psychological effects of severe burn injuries. Psychol Bull 1993;113(2):362–78.
4. Patterson DR, Jensen M. Hypnosis and clinical pain. Psychol Bull 2003;129(4):495–521.

5. Patterson DR, Finch CP, Wiechman SA, et al. Premorbid mental health status of adult burn patients: comparison with a normative sample. J Burn Care Rehabil 2003;24(5):347–50.
6. Patterson DR, Tininenko J, Ptacek JT. Pain during burn hospitalization predicts long-term outcome. J Burn Care Res 2006;27(5):719–26.
7. Noronha DO, Faust J. Identifying the variables impacting post-burn psychological adjustment: a meta-analysis. J Pediatr Psychol 2007;32(3):380–91.
8. Ptacek JT, Patterson DR, Montgomery BK, et al. Pain, coping, and adjustment in patients with severe burns: preliminary findings from a prospective study. J Pain Symptom Manage 1995;10:446–55.
9. Wiechman SA, Ptacek JT, Patterson DR, et al. Rates, trends, and depression following burn injuries. J Burn Care Rehabil 2001;22(6):417–24.
10. Lazarus RS, Folkman S. Stress, appraisal and coping. New York: Springer; 1984.
11. Taylor SE, Stanton AL. Coping resources, coping processes, and mental health. Annu Rev Clin Psychol 2007;3:377–401.
12. Suls J, Fletcher B. The relative efficacy of avoidant and nonavoidant coping strategies: a meta-analysis. Health Psychol 1985;4(3):249–88.
13. Stanton AL, Revenson TA, Tennen H. Health psychology: psychological adjustment to chronic disease. Annu Rev Psychol 2007;58:565–92.
14. Folkman S, Lazarus RS. An analysis of coping in a middle-aged community sample. J Health Soc Behav 1980;21:219–39.
15. Fauerbach J, Lawrence J, Haythornthwaite J, et al. Psychiatric history affects post trauma morbidity in a burn injured adult sample. Psychosomatics 1997; 38:374–85.
16. Fauerbach JA, McKibben J, Bienvenu OJ, et al. Psychological distress after major burn injury. Psychosom Med 2007;69(5):473–82.
17. Edwards RR, Magyar-Russell G, Thombs B, et al. Acute pain at discharge from hospitalization is a prospective predictor of long-term suicidal ideation after burn injury. Arch Phys Med Rehabil 2007;88(12 Suppl 2):S36–42.
18. Ullrich PM, Askay SW, Patterson DR. Pain, depression, and physical functioning following burn injury. Rehabil Psychol 2009;54(2):211–6.
19. Fukunishi I. Relationship of cosmetic disfigurement to the severity of posttraumatic stress disorder in burn injury or digital amputation. Psychother Psychosom 1999;68(2):82–6.
20. Madianos MG, Papaghelis M, Ioannovich J, et al. Psychiatric disorders in burn patients: a follow-up study. Psychother Psychosom 2001;70(1):30–7.
21. Ptacek J, Patterson D, Heimbach D. Inpatient depression in persons with burns. J Burn Care Rehabil 2002;23(1):1–9.
22. Tedstone JE, Tarrier N. An investigation of the prevalence of psychological morbidity in burn-injured patients. Burns 1997;23(7/8):550–4.
23. Williams EE, Griffiths TA. Psychological consequences of burn injury. Burns 1991;17(6):478–80.
24. Bauer K, Hardy P, Van Sorsten V. Posttraumatic stress disorder in burn populations: a critical review of the literature. J Burn Care Rehabil 1998;19:230–40.
25. Ehde D, Patterson D, Wiechman S, et al. Post-traumatic stress symptoms and distress one year after burn injury. J Burn Care Rehabil 2000;21(2):105–11.
26. Boeve SA, Aaron LA, Martin-Herz SP, et al. Sleep disturbance after burn injury. J Burn Care Rehabil 2002;23(1):32–8.
27. Lawrence J, Fauerbach J, Eudell E, et al. Sleep disturbance following burn injury: a frequent yet understudied complication. J Burn Care Rehabil 1998; 19:480–6.

28. Jaffe S, Patterson DR. Treating sleep problems in patients with burn injuries: practical considerations. J Burn Care Rehabil 2004;25(3):294–305.
29. Fauerbach JA, Heinberg LJ, Lawrence JW, et al. Effect of early body image dissatisfaction on subsequent psychological and physical adjustment after disfiguring injury. Psychosom Med 2000;62(4):576–82.
30. Bianchi TL. Aspects of sexuality after burn injury: outcomes in men. J Burn Care Rehabil 1997;18(2):183–6 [discussion: 182].
31. Wiechman Askay SA, Patterson DR. Psychological rehabilitation in burn injuries. In: Frank RG, Rosenthal M, Caplan B, editors. Handbook of rehabilitation psychology. 2nd edition. Washington, DC: American Psychological Association; 2009. p. 107–18.
32. Fauerbach JA, Lawrence JW, Munster AM, et al. Prolonged adjustment difficulties among those with acute posttrauma distress following burn injury. J Behav Med 1999;22(4):359–78.
33. Patterson DR, Ptacek JT, Cromes F, et al. The 2000 clinical research award: describing and predicting distress and satisfaction with life for burn survivors. J Burn Care Rehabil 2000;21(6):490–8.
34. Difede J, Ptacek JT, Roberts J, et al. Acute stress disorder after burn injury: a predictor of posttraumatic stress disorder? Psychosom Med 2002;64(5):826–34.
35. Bryant R. Predictors of post-traumatic stress disorder following burn injury. Burns 1996;22:89–92.
36. Fleming MP, Difede J. Effects of varying scoring rules of the Clinician Administered PTSD Scale (CAPS) for the diagnosis of PTSD after acute burn injury. J Trauma Stress 1999;12(3):535–42.
37. Lambert JF, Difede J, Contrada RJ. The relationship of attribution of responsibility to acute stress disorder among hospitalized burn patients. J Nerv Ment Dis 2004;192(4):304–12.
38. Ehde DM, Patterson DR, Wiechman SA, et al. Post-traumatic stress symptoms and distress following acute burn injury. Burns 1999;25:587–92.
39. Van Loey NE, Maas CJ, Faber AW, et al. Predictors of chronic posttraumatic stress symptoms following burn injury: results of a longitudinal study. J Trauma Stress 2003;16(4):361–9.
40. El hamaoui Y, Yaalaoui S, Chihabeddine K, et al. Post-traumatic stress disorder in burned patients. Burns 2002;28(7):647–50.
41. Difede J, Barocas D. Acute intrusive and avoidant PTSD symptoms as predictors of chronic PTSD following burn injury. J Trauma Stress 1999;12(2):363–9.
42. American Psychiatric Association. Diagnostic and statistical manual of mental disorders. 4th edition. Washington, DC: American Psychiatric Association; 1994.
43. McKibben JB, Bresnick MG, Wiechman Askay SA, et al. Acute stress disorder and posttraumatic stress disorder: a prospective study of prevalence, course, and predictors in a sample with major burn injuries. J Burn Care Res 2008; 29(1):22–35.
44. Weathers F, Litz B, Herman D, et al. The PTSD Checklist (PCL): reliability, validity, and diagnostic utility. Paper presented at the Annual convention of the international society for traumatic stress studies. San Antonio (TX), October, 1993.
45. Thombs BD, Bresnick MG, Magyar-Russell G. Depression in survivors of burn injury: a systematic review. Gen Hosp Psychiatry 2006;28(6):494–502.
46. Thombs BD, Bass EB, Ford DE, et al. Prevalence of depression in survivors of acute myocardial infarction. J Gen Intern Med 2006;21(1):30–8.
47. Zigmond AS, Snaith RP. The hospital anxiety and depression scale. Acta Psychiatr Scand 1983;67(6):361–70.

48. Beck A, Steer RA, Brown G. BDI-II manual. 2nd edition. San Antonio (TX): The Psychological Corporation; 1996.
49. Perry S, Heidrich G. Management of pain during debridement: a survey of U.S. burn units. Pain 1982;13(3):267–80.
50. Choiniere M, Melzack R, Rondeau J, et al. The pain of burns: characteristics and correlates. J Trauma 1989;29(11):1531–9.
51. Patterson DR, Sharar SR. Burn pain. In: Loeser JD, Butler SH, Chapman CR, et al, editors. Bonica's management of pain. 3rd edition. Philadelphia: Lippincott; 2001. p. 780–7.
52. Malenfant A, Forget R, Amsel R, et al. Tactile, thermal and pain sensibility in burned patients with and without chronic pain and paresthesia problems. Pain 1998;77(3):241–51.
53. Choiniere M, Melzack R, Papillon J. Pain and paresthesia in patients with healed burns: an exploratory study. J Pain Symptom Manage 1991;6:437–44.
54. Schneider JC, Harris NL, El Shami A, et al. A descriptive review of neuropathic-like pain after burn injury. J Burn Care Res 2006;27(4):524–8.
55. Dauber A, Osgood PF, Breslau AJ, et al. Chronic persistent pain after severe burns: a survey of 358 burn survivors. Pain Med 2002;3(1):6–17.
56. Porter J, Jick H. Addiction rare in patients treated with narcotics. N Engl J Med 1980;302(2):123.
57. Faucher L, Furukwaw K. Practice guidelines for the management of pain. J Burn Care Rehabil 2006;27(5):659–68.
58. Summer GJ, Puntillo KA, Miaskowski C, et al. Burn injury pain: the continuing challenge. J Pain 2007;8(7):533–48.
59. Martin-Herz SP, Thurber CA, Patterson DR. Psychological principles of burn wound pain in children. II: treatment applications. J Burn Care Rehabil 2000; 21(5):458–72 [discussion: 457].
60. Patterson DR, Tininenko JR, Schmidt AE, et al. Virtual reality hypnosis: a case report. Int J Clin Exp Hypn 2004;52(1):27–38.
61. Hoffman HG, Patterson DR, Carrougher GJ, et al. Effectiveness of virtual reality-based pain control with multiple treatments. Clin J Pain 2001;17(3): 229–35.
62. Kahneman D. Attention and effort. Englewood Cliffs (NJ): Prentice-Hall; 1973.
63. Shiffrin R, Schneider W. Controlled and automatic human information processing. II: perceptual learning, automatic attending, and a general theory. Psychol Rev 1977;84:127–90.
64. Hoffman HG. Role of memory strength in reality monitoring decisions: evidence from source attribution bias. J Exp Psychol Learn Mem Cogn 1997;23(2): 371–83.
65. Hoffman HG, Doctor JN, Patterson DR, et al. Use of virtual reality as an adjunctive treatment of adolescent burn pain during wound care: a case report. Pain 2000;85:305–9.
66. Hoffman HG, Patterson DR, Carrougher GJ. Use of virtual reality for adjunctive treatment of adult burn pain during physical therapy: a controlled study. Clin J Pain 2000;16:244–50.
67. Hoffman HG, Patterson DR, Carrougher GJ, et al. The effectiveness of virtual reality pain control with multiple treatments of longer durations: a case study. Int J Hum Comput Interact 2001;13:1–12.
68. Barber J. A brief introduction to hypnotic analgesia. In: Barber J, editor. Hypnosis and suggestion in the treatment of pain. A clinical guide. New York: W.W. Norton & Company; 1996. p. 3–33.

69. Patterson DR. Burn pain. In: Barber J, editor. Hypnosis and suggestion in the treatment of pain. New York: W.W. Norton & Company; 1996. p. 267–302.

70. Barber J. Rapid induction analgesia: a clinical report. Am J Clin Hypn 1977;19: 138–47.

71. Greenberg JS. Comprehensive stress management. Dubuque (IA): Bron & Benchmark; 1993.

72. Jacobson E. Progressive relaxation. Chicago: University of Chicago Press; 1938.

73. Ehde DM, Patterson DR, Fordyce WE. The quota system in burn rehabilitation. J Burn Care Rehabil 1998;19(5):436–40.

74. Holzman AD, Turk DC. Pain management. Oxford (UK): Pergamon Press; 1986.

75. Turk DC, Meichenbaum D, Genest M. Pain and behavioral medicine: a cognitive-behavioral perspective. New York: Guilford Press; 1983.

76. Langer E, Janis I, Wolfer J. Reduction of psychological stress in surgical patients. J Exp Soc Psychol 1975;11:165–9.

77. Thurber CA, Martin-Herz SP, Patterson DR. Psychological principles of burn wound pain in children. I: theoretical framework. J Burn Care Rehabil 2000; 21(4):376–87 [discussion: 375].

78. Everett J, Patterson DR, Chen AC. Cognitive and behavioral treatments for burn pain. Pain Clin 1990;3:1133–45.

79. Zeltzer L. Pain and symptom management. In: Bearson DJ, Mullhern RK, editors. Pediatric psychooncology: psychological perspectives on children with cancer. New York: Oxford University Press; 1994. p. 61–83.

80. Fordyce WE. Behavioral methods for chronic pain and illness. St Louis (MO): C.V. Mosby; 1976.

81. Hanson MD, Gauld M, Wathen CN, et al. Nonpharmacological interventions for acute wound care distress in pediatric patients with burn injury: a systematic review. J Burn Care Res 2008;5:730–41.

82. Foertsch CE, O'Hara MW, Stroddard FJ, et al. Treatment-resistant pain and distress during pediatric burn dressing changes. J Burn Care Rehabil 1998; 19:219–24.

83. de Jong AEE, Middlekoop E, Faber AW, et al. Nonpharmacological nursing interventions for procedural pain relief in adults with burns: a systematic literature review. Burns 2007;33:811–27.

84. Ancoli-Israel S, Roth T. Characteristics of insomnia in the United States: results of the 1991 national sleep foundation survey I. Sleep 1999;22(2):S347–53.

85. Chesson A, Hartse K, Anderson W, et al. Practice parameters for the evaluation of chronic insomnia. An American Academy of Sleep Medicine report. Standards of Practice Committee of the American Academy of Sleep Medicine. Sleep 2000;23(2):237–41.

86. Weyerer S, Dilling H. Prevalence and treatment of insomnia in the community: results from the Upper Bavarian Field Study. Sleep 1991;14(5):392–8.

87. Rose M, Sanford A, Thomas C, et al. Factors altering the sleep of burned children. Sleep 2001;24(1):45–51.

88. Kravitz M, McCoy BJ, Tompkins DM, et al. Sleep disorders in children after burn injury. J Burn Care Rehabil 1993;14(1):83–90.

89. Gottschlich MM, Jenkins M, Mayes T, et al. Lack of effect of sleep on energy expenditure and physiologic measures in critically ill burn patients. J Am Diet Assoc 1997;97(2):131–9.

90. Gottschlich MM, Jenkins ME, Mayes T, et al. The 1994 clinical research award. A prospective clinical study of the polysomnographic stages of sleep after burn injury. J Burn Care Rehabil 1994;15(6):486–92.

91. Robertson CF, Zuker R, Dabrowski B, et al. Obstructive sleep apnea: a complication of burns to the head and neck in children. J Burn Care Rehabil 1985;6(4): 353–7.
92. Ahee AM, Smith SJ, Pliska-Matyshak G, et al. When does itching start and stop post-burn? J Burn Care Rehabil 1999;20(1 Pt 2):S187.
93. Goutos I, Dziewulski P, Richardson PM. Pruritus in burns: review article. J Burn Care Res 2009;30(2):221–8.
94. Bell PL, Gabriel V. Evidence based review for the treatment of post-burn pruritus. J Burn Care Res 2009;30(1):55–61.
95. Gibran NS. Practice Guidelines for burn care, 2006. J Burn Care Res 2006; 27(4):437–8.
96. Allison KP, Kiernan MN, Waters RA, et al. Pulsed dye laser treatment of burn scars. Alleviation or irritation? Burns 2003;29(3):207–13.
97. Baker RA, Zeller RA, Klein RL, et al. Burn wound itch control using H1 and H2 antagonists. J Burn Care Rehabil 2001;22(4):263–8.
98. Fauerbach JA, Heinberg LJ, Lawrence JW, et al. Coping with body image changes following a disfiguring burn injury. Health Psychol 2002;21(2):115–21.
99. Lawrence JW, Fauerbach JA, Heinberg L, et al. Visible vs hidden scars and their relation to body esteem. J Burn Care Rehabil 2004;25(1):25–32.
100. Abdullah A, Blakeney P, Hunt R, et al. Visible scars and self-esteem in pediatric patients with burns. J Burn Care Rehabil 1994;15(2):164–8.
101. Pruzinsky T, Cash TF. Integrative themes in body-image development, deviance, and change. In: Cash TF, Pruzinsky T, editors. Body images: development, deviance, and change. New York: Guilford Press; 1990. p. 337–49.
102. Partridge J. When burns affect the way you look. London: Changing Faces; 1997.
103. Kammerer B. BEST program provides key to successful community reintegration. Burn Support News 2010;1:1–4.
104. Williams RM, Patterson DR, Schwenn C, et al. Evaluation of a peer consultation program for burn inpatients. 2000 ABA paper. J Burn Care Rehabil 2002;23(6): 449–53.

Exercise Following Burn Injury

Barbara J. de Lateur, MD, MS[a], Wendy S. Shore, PhD[b],*

KEYWORDS

• Burn injury • Exercise • Rehabilitation

A major barrier to return to work and full community reintegration for burned individuals is fatigue, a highly prevalent symptom. In an effort to determine the origin of this fatigue, a study of outcomes, in various domains, was conducted at Harborview Medical Center in Seattle on more than 100 survivors of major burns who had been hospitalized for 1 day or more (average length of stay 15 days) and age- and sex-matched, unburned controls. Data were collected that measured the strength and the relative endurance ratio of individual muscles, such as the quadriceps. (The relative endurance ratio is the ratio of the value of peak torque in the last of a series of contractions to the value of peak torque in the first contraction. Since the units of measure cancel out in this ratio, the result is a unit-free number.) Somewhat surprisingly, this ratio (approximately 0.7) was the same, on average, in the burned subjects as in the age- and sex-matched controls. The difference was in the strength of the subjects with burns, who were much weaker than the controls. This weakness applied to all muscles tested, regardless of whether there was a burn in the region of the given muscle or not; however, a burn in the region was associated with greater weakness. The strength of subjects with burns approached, as a limit, the strength of the controls, only at 2 years postburn.[1] The common complaint of fatigue most likely resulted from the muscular weakness, which caused the subjects to operate at a higher percent maximal effort, even for their usual activities.

Another, more recent, study found that patients with severe burns (>30% total body surface area) had weaker muscles even years (15–92 months) after the burn injury, suggesting either inability to fully recover muscle strength or insufficient rehabilitation. Interestingly, patients with less than 30% total body surface area showed no difference compared with controls.[2]

In an ongoing study of the effects of an augmented exercise program by de Lateur and colleagues[3] (plus as-yet unpublished observations), some postburn subjects,

The authors have nothing to disclose.
a Department of Physical Medicine and Rehabilitation, Johns Hopkins Medical Institutions, AA Building, Room 1654, 4940 Eastern Avenue, Baltimore, MD 21224-2780, USA
b Department of Physical Medicine and Rehabilitation, Johns Hopkins Medical Institutions, 92 North Broadway, Suite 413, Baltimore, MD 21239, USA
* Corresponding author.
E-mail address: Wshore1@jhmi.edu

Phys Med Rehabil Clin N Am 22 (2011) 347–350
doi:10.1016/j.pmr.2011.02.003
1047-9651/11/$ – see front matter © 2011 Elsevier Inc. All rights reserved.

independently ambulatory and able to walk on a treadmill, have very low baseline maximal aerobic capacities. In some of these, the values are so low (approximately 11 mL/kg/min) that if they were frail elderly subjects, they would be classified as fitting into a group considered to be unable to live independently in the community (the burned subjects were younger and were, in fact, living independently).

Muscle wasting (catabolism) and hypermetabolism are prevalent in adult[4] and pediatric[5] burn survivors. In a study of severely burned children, hypermetabolism and catabolism remain elevated for at least 9 months after injury.

The work of Alloju and colleagues[6] has shown that severely burned children, compared with nonburned children, had significantly lower lean body mass and lower peak torque, as well as total work performance at 6 months post burn. These investigators, and Pereira and colleagues,[5] comment on the hypermetabolic response to thermal injury and its marked catabolic effect. It is likely that this hypermetabolic response and its catabolism is the cause of muscle weakness.

THE NATURAL COURSE

The studies cited above indicate that a slow return to normal or near-normal muscle strength (at 2 years postburn) is the natural course of recovery. With no special interventions, other than the "usual care" tailored to the needs of the individual, postburn patients will make gradual improvement in strength[1] and aerobic capacity[3]; although, in the latter case, the improvement may not reach statistical significance. This is in marked contrast to the intervention group (usual care plus an augmented 12-week exercise program), which had a robust improvement in aerobic capacity.

HOW SHOULD ONE DEVELOP A PROGRAM FOR PATIENTS AFTER A BURN INJURY?

Hart and colleagues[7] have suggested that because there is substantial evidence that catabolic and metabolic responses to severe burn injuries linger many months after the injury, therapeutic attempts to address the catabolic and hypermetabolic response to severe injury should also be continued long after injury. There is little question that burn patients cannot only tolerate activity, they greatly benefit from it.[8–10]

In the initial phase, when the patient is in a catabolic state, the targeted physical and occupational therapies, with a gentle aerobic program, may be as much as the patient can tolerate. This rest of this article is devoted to exercise interventions for the patient well enough to be discharged to the community.

SPECIFICITY VERSUS GENERALIZABILITY: THE PRINCIPLE OF INITIAL CONDITION

The principle of initial condition asserts that the worse the initial condition (barring a neuropathy or flexion contractures), the greater the response to exercise intervention and the more the response can be generalized. For example, in a study of frail elders, exercise on a treadmill, an aerobic intervention, resulted in increased strength.[3,11] Likewise, one could predict up to 49% of the variance of treadmill performance by the relative strength (strength-to-weight-to-height ratio) of certain lower-body muscles. This seems counterintuitive because the aerobic and strength systems are so different. It is commonly understood that one should train for the specific task, such as resistance training for weight lifting and running sprints for track competitions. Indeed, in highly trained athletes, it is important to train on the performance task. However, in postburn patients, the principle of initial condition works in the patient's favor and permits a number of options for exercise interventions, determined by patient preference and equipment availability. The therapist or trainer can be confident of increased strength, as well as aerobic performance, in response to treadmill or stationary bicycle exercise.

HOW DOES ONE GO ABOUT IT?

There are many standard programs available, such as the DeLorme[12] or the Oxford[13] progressive resistive exercise programs. However, to avoid injury, or even an unpleasant experience, which might prompt the patient to discontinue the program, the authors suggest a very gradually progressive program, determined by the performance in a baseline work-to-tolerance period. An example is a very deconditioned person, with little or no recent experience with a regular exercise program and no equipment. This person could be asked to keep a record of minutes walked, for the sake of walking each day for 10 days. At the end of those 10 days, an average number of minutes walked would be found, being sure to include any zero-minute days. Ten percent of that average could be subtracted, and the resultant number would provide the quota for the daily minutes to be walked for the first week. Each week another minute would be added to the daily quota. Thus, if the baseline average was 10 minutes, the quota for the first week would be a daily walk of 9 minutes, the second week 10 minutes, the third 11 minutes, and so forth. The patient should keep a daily record, so that the person (physician, therapist, trainer) following him or her can check this. From a behavioral point of view, the physician (therapist, trainer) should show a high degree of enthusiasm and praise for the patient following this quota faithfully. The walking can be capped off at 30 minutes, as long as it is done every day, without fail, just as one would ordinarily not skip the daily shower.

HOW LONG?

The typical exercise study is performed for 12 weeks (or, in some cases, 10 weeks). This is not a biological number. Rather, it is most often a period of convenience, such as the length of an academic quarter or semester, because many of the early exercise studies were performed on college students. This length of time is unlikely to be sufficient in the gradually progressive walking program for an extremely deconditioned subject, such as the example given above, and it should be extended beyond 12 weeks. If the subject's initial condition permitted a vigorous progressive resistive exercise program, such as the DeLorme or Oxford techniques, three or four times a week, it should be sufficient. After the rehabilitation period, The American College of Sports Medicine's guidelines indicate that shifting to a twice-a-week weight-training program is sufficient for maintenance. In addition, moderate aerobic activity should be continued at least 5 days a week.[14]

HOW FIT? FIT FOR WHAT?

The word "fit" itself implies fit for something. In this case, if the patient can resume his or her usual activities, including bathing, dressing, household duties, work, recreation, and travel, then she or he can be considered to have a baseline level of fitness. It is important to note, however, that if no more activity than performance of activities of daily living is the norm, the individual will gradually lose both muscle mass and aerobic endurance, eventually ending up back in the "frail" category. The minimal activity recommendations from the American College of Sports Medicine, given above, are necessary for long-term ability to function independently. If the patient wishes to go beyond those guidelines, then more vigorous weight training of individual muscles, as well as treadmill, elliptical, and other aerobic practices should be employed, just as in the case of persons never burned.

SOME PRECAUTIONS

Care should be taken in the case of impaired sensation (as in nerve entrapment) or grafted areas underneath shoes. The patient should be taught to inspect his or her skin after each exercise session and adjust the type or the duration of the exercise accordingly. As mentioned above, the generalizability of early exercise in very deconditioned patients permits options that avoid skin injury.

REFERENCES

1. de Lateur BJ, Giaconi RM, Alquist AD. Fatigue and performance: data from normal adults, and from patients with neuromuscular and musculoskeletal syndromes; response to training. Proceedings AAEE Diagnostic Program, Thirty-fifth Annual Meeting; 1988.
2. St-Pierre DM, Choiniere M, Forget R, et al. Muscle strength in individuals with healed burns. Arch Phys Med Rehabil 1998;79(2):155–61.
3. de Lateur BJ, Magyar-Russell G, Bresnick MG, et al. Augmented exercise in the treatment of deconditioning from major burn injury. Arch Phys Med Rehabil 2007; 88(12 Suppl 2):S18–23.
4. Hasselgren PO. Burns and metabolism. J Am Coll Surg 1999;188(2):98–103.
5. Pereira C, Murphy K, Jeschke M, et al. Post burn muscle wasting and the effects of treatments. Int J Biochem Cell Biol 2005;37(10):1948–61.
6. Alloju SM, Herndon DN, McEntire SJ, et al. Assessment of muscle function in severely burned children. Burns 2008;34(4):452–9.
7. Hart DW, Wolf SE, Mlcak R, et al. Persistence of muscle catabolism after severe burn. Surgery 2000;128(2):312–9.
8. McEntire SJ, Herndon DN, Sanford AP, et al. Thermoregulation during exercise in severely burned children. Pediatr Rehabil 2006;9(1):57–64.
9. Suman OE, Mlcak RP, Herndon DN. Effect of exercise training on pulmonary function in children with thermal injury. J Burn Care Rehabil 2002;23(4):288–93 [discussion: 287].
10. Whitney JD, Parkman S. The effect of early postoperative physical activity on tissue oxygen and wound healing. Biol Res Nurs 2004;6(2):79–89.
11. Buchner DM, Cress ME, Wagner EH, et al. The Seattle FICSIT/MoveIt study: the effect of exercise on gait and balance in older adults. J Am Geriatr Soc 1993; 41(3):321–5.
12. DeLorme TL, Watkins AL. Techniques of progressive resistance exercise. Arch Phys Med Rehabil 1948;29(5):263–73.
13. Zinovieff AN. Heavy-resistance exercises the "Oxford Technique". Br J Phys Med 1951;14(6):129–32.
14. Haskell WL, Lee IM, Pate RR, et al. Physical activity and public health: updated recommendation for adults from the American College of Sports Medicine and the American Heart Association. Med Sci Sports Exerc 2007;39(8):1423–34.

Community Integration Outcome After Burn Injury

Peter C. Esselman, MD

KEYWORDS

- Burn injury • Community integration • Rehabilitation
- Vocational rehabilitation

The goal of a burn rehabilitation program over the long term is to maximize function and increase participation in the community, including return to work or school. To examine factors that have an impact on return to previous activities, it is important to have a model that incorporates the many complex issues involved. The World Health Organization has developed a model in the International Classification of Functioning, Disability and Health (ICF). The ICF is a biopsychosocial model of disease that incorporates all aspects of function and disability. It is not focused on the etiology of the injury but on the loss of function that occurs as a result of the injury and the impact on participation. In addition, the ICF is a model that has broad utility across diverse environments and communities because it is not based on single individuals but on the context of the loss of function in the social community.[1,2]

In the context of burn injury, the ICF model characterizes the injury in regards to the anatomic body structure, such as an injury to the skin or other structure. Body function is described in terms of the impact of changes on the physiologic function of the skin and other structures. An example is an inability to move through a normal range of joint motion due to scarring. Activities are described as the execution of a task or action, such as ambulation and dressing tasks. Participation is the involvement in a life situation, such as work and school but also leisure and social activities. The ICF model also acknowledges the important impact and influence of environmental factors, such as age, gender, and coping style, that have an impact on long-term outcome. In the case of burn injuries, important personal factors include an individual's reaction to changes in body image along with the environmental factors regarding the attitude and response of others to visible scars.[3]

This work was supported by funds from the National Institute on Disability and Rehabilitation Research in the Office of Special Education and Rehabilitative Services in the U.S. Department of Education.

Department of Rehabilitation Medicine, University of Washington Burn Center, Harborview Medical Center, University of Washington, 325 9th Avenue, Box 359612, Seattle, WA 98104, USA

E-mail address: esselman@u.washington.edu

The framework of the ICF has been utilized to examine outcomes after burn injuries.[4,5] Falder and colleagues[4] established 7 core domains of assessment important to the outcome of individuals with burn injuries. The domains are (1) skin, (2) neuromuscular function, (3) sensory function and pain, (4) psychological function, (5) physical role function, (6) community participation, and (7) perceived quality of life. The ICF classification model should be used for future evaluation and development of tools to measure outcome after burn injury. The importance of the ICF is that it recognizes individual factors along with environmental factors in the model. This article focuses on participation after burn injury, with a focus on factors that have an impact on a person's ability to return to work or school.

RETURN TO WORK

Often, the long-term goal of a burn rehabilitation program is return to work because this indicates an achievement of significant community participation. In a multicenter study, Brych and colleagues[6] determined that among individuals with burn injuries who were employed outside of the home at the time of their burn injury, the average time off work was 17 weeks. The study reports that 66% of the subjects were employed at the 6-month follow-up and 90% had returned to work at 2 years after the burn injury. In other studies, between 60% and 80% of individuals returned to work at 1 year after injury.[7–9] In a study of soldiers with burn injuries sustained in Operation Enduring Freedom/Operation Iraqi Freedom, 67% were able to return to military duty and 33% were discharged from the military due to their injuries.[10]

An important personal factor that influences community participation, such as employment after a burn injury, is the employment status of the individual at the time of the burn injury. In a multicenter study of 770 individuals admitted to a burn center with severe burn injuries (average total body surface area [TBSA] 20.2%), Fauerbach and colleagues[11] reported that only 70% of the patients were employed outside of the home at the time of their burn injury. They also noted that of the employed group, 42% sustained their injury at work. The study reports that those individuals who were not employed at the time of injury had significantly higher levels of history of pre-existing disability, medical problems, and history of psychological problems and were more likely to have a positive toxicology screen for alcohol at the time of the injury. Individuals who were employed at the time of injury were more likely to have sustained a hand burn and require hand surgery. Individuals not employed were more likely to sustain an inhalation injury. This is consistent with the likely mechanism of injury. Individuals who are employed are more likely to be injured at work in an open space or factory where they are less likely to sustain an inhalation injury, but their hands are more exposed to a heat source and more likely to be burned. Individuals burned in a nonwork setting, such as at home or in a vehicle, are more likely to sustain an inhalation injury. This study points out the personal factors (employment, preinjury disability, and psychological issues) that can have an impact on long-term outcome.

Several studies have identified burn injury–related and other factors that predict return to work. Many studies identify indicators of burn injury severity (percentage TBSA, length of hospitalization, and length of ICU stay) as predictors of not returning to work.[6,12] An inhalation injury is another injury characteristic found to limit return to previous activities.[10] In many patients, hand burns are a factor limiting the ability to return to work,[9] but in a study of injured soldiers, the presence of a hand burn was not a significant predictor of the ability to return to military duty.[10] As indicated in the ICF model, there are many environmental and personal factors that influence participation after a burn injury. In a study of 225 individuals with severe burn injuries admitted to the University of Alabama burn center, injury severity indicators were not significantly related to employment.[13] The variables that increased the probability of employment after a burn injury were being white race, not blaming oneself, receiving workman's compensation, and being employed before the injury.[13] Preinjury employment status was a significant predictor of postinjury employment and this was seen other studies.[9,12] In a study by Schneider and colleagues,[8] significant predictors of being disabled longer than 12 months included length of hospitalization, receiving inpatient rehabilitation, burn injury occurring at work, and an electrical injury as the etiology of injury.

Brych and colleagues[6] reported that at 6 months and 24 months after injury, a psychiatric history significantly reduced the odds of returning to work. Postinjury psychological issues are also associated with work status. Studies from Sweden have studied individuals years after burn injuries and reported that predictors of employment include burn-related factors and personality-related factors.[14,15] Individuals not working demonstrated worse psychosocial health, such as greater fear avoidance and posttraumatic stress symptoms, compared with those employed. Those unemployed also reported a lower health-related quality of life compared with those working. Chronic pain is also a common problem that limits employment and quality of life. In one study, pain was reported in 60% of the unemployed group and in only 18% of those working.[14]

Several studies have looked in detail at specific barriers to returning to work after a burn injury. In one study of patient self-reported barriers to returning to work, physical abilities, working conditions, and wound issues were important factors within the first few months after the burn injury. In those individuals with longer-term disability who had not returned to work within 6 months after the injury, psychological and social factors were more important barriers. These included barriers, such as concern about appearance and working with others, being afraid to leave home or being afraid of the workplace, and depressed mood.[7] In another study, review of medical records showed that the most common reported barriers to return to work included pain, neurologic problems, impaired mobility, and psychiatric issues.[8] A study from Sweden identified facilitators and barriers to return to work through interviews of individuals who had sustained burn injuries at an average of 4.6 years prior to the study.[16] To a large degree, facilitators were individual characteristics, such as being able to set up goals in rehabilitation, being persistent, having willpower, and the individuals' own ability to take action. Support from individuals' families and social network were identified as important facilitators. Identified barriers to returning to work included the lack of an individualized rehabilitation plan and lack of psychological support. Physical impairments, such as pain, wound issues, and strength, were barriers early in the rehabilitation but not considered significant long-term barriers to return to work.[16]

Return to work after severe burn injuries is a complex interaction of factors involving injury severity, personal characteristics, work-related issues, social support, and medical and rehabilitation treatment. In a qualitative research study that examined patient characteristics in relation to employment status, Mackay and colleagues[17] placed patients in 5 categories: (1) defeated, (2) burdened, (3) affected, (4) unchanged, and (5) stronger. The defeated group was characterized by history of manual labor, injury at work, fear of the workplace, symptoms of depression, and being unsuccessful in attempts to return to work. The burdened group was unemployed prior to their injury and the physical and psychological impact of the burn injury compounded their previous problems. The affected group returned to work but struggled with physical and psychological issues, making stable employment challenging. The unchanged group returned to the same job and often benefited from a supportive employer. The stronger group returned to the same or different job, had strong social support, and found strength from their personality.[17]

Individuals with electrical injuries often have challenges returning to work. One confounding factor is that electrical injuries are more likely to occur at the workplace. In one study, 91% of electrical injuries were work related. In long-term follow-up, 23% returned to the same work duties, 45% changed duties, and 32% remained unemployed.[18] There are high rates of neuropsychiatric issues reported after electrical injuries that have an impact on a person's ability to return to work. In addition, patients sustaining electrical injuries on the job are often afraid to return to the workplace. These problems are reported in both high-voltage and low-voltage electrical injuries.[19,20]

In the treatment of burn injuries, it is important to have a coordinated medical team skilled in acute management and long-term rehabilitation of individuals with severe burn injuries. It is appropriate that treatment focus on the important issues of wound care, preventing scarring and contractures and improving function. But, it is equally important that treatment focus on other factors that influence an individual's ability to return to participation in the community, including return to work. In several studies, psychological issues have been found to be important in returning to work. Therefore, it is important for patients to have access to psychological treatment during the acute phase after burn injury and during the longer rehabilitation treatment. It is also important for many patients to have the assistance of a vocational rehabilitation counselor. In a study by Öster and colleagues,[16] facilitators to return to work included the ability to have modified work duties, a change in workplace, or an alteration in work hours. Having a supportive employer and coworkers was also identified as a facilitator to returning to work. A vocational rehabilitation counselor can coordinate a return to work plan with the injured worker and the employer. The goal is that the return to work plan be structured to optimize success. A patient who returns to full-duty employment too soon without an assessment of the physical and psychological demands may be unsuccessful, leading to long-term disability. A well-planned return to work with modified work duties or hours, coordinated with a supportive employer, can lead to a permanent return to work.

RETURN TO SCHOOL

In the pediatric population with burn injuries, it is important to focus on the transition back to school. In a study by Staley and colleagues,[21] children admitted with burn injuries, with an average of 25.9% TBSA burn, returned to school, on average, fewer than 8 days after discharge from the hospital. In this study, 34% of the children had an in-person school reentry visit by a member of the burn team, and, in cases in which a school visit was not possible, the transition back to school was facilitated by a phone call or educational materials provided to the school. Another study reported similar data, with an average time of return to school of 10.5 days after hospital discharge.[22] The only predictors of delayed return to school were hospital length of stay, male gender, and older age.[22]

Although a school visit may be the optimal way to transition a child back to the classroom, the location of regional burn centers and the distance involved makes such a visit challenging. Blakeney and colleagues[23] report on the use of individualized video to assist with the transition in patients with severe burn injuries. In this report, a video was made if the burn injury was greater than 40% TBSA or involved the hands or face. The video explains the burn injury, hospital care, scarring after a burn injury, and any garments or splints the child may be wearing. The video can explain any changes in physical abilities or appearance. The patients are encouraged to talk on the video to provide their own perspective. The video is then provided to the school prior to the child's return. This video or in-person visit was a highly valuable resource by teachers and parents for facilitating the return of the patient to school. This study reports that the most difficult aspects of adjustment for students as reported by the parents was confronting the reactions of others and accepting physical limitations. Parents reported that these concerns primarily occurred outside of the school setting, possibly due to the structured school reentry program and preparation of the teachers and fellow students.[23]

The Phoenix Society for Burn Survivors has developed a comprehensive manual to assist burn centers in facilitating the transition of children back to school. The goals of the reentry program are to educate school faculty and students regarding a student's story and injuries, encourage empathy, provide tools for the student with a burn injury to encourage positive coping techniques and socialization, and teach classmates appropriate and positive ways to interact with the student.[24] Identification of a school reentry coordinator is important for the success of the program. The school reentry coordinator can contact the school and coordinate a school presentation if indicated. A school presentation provides information about the injuries and gives advice to the students in school regarding how to interact with a student with a burn injury on return to school. The coordinator can also work with the student and family to facilitate a successful transition back to school.[24]

SUMMARY

It is important to focus on community integration, including return to work and school, early during treatment after burn injuries. A careful analysis of the potential barriers to return to activities can help focus a treatment team and provide appropriate support for a return to work or school plan. Psychological intervention is often an important component of a return to work or school plan. Vocational rehabilitation counselors and school reentry coordinators are valuable assets to coordinating with a treatment team and communicating with a workplace or school. A successful return to work or school is often achieved with a coordinated and supportive approach.

REFERENCES

1. World Health Organization. International classification of functioning, disability and health: ICF. Geneva (IL): WHO; 2001.
2. Stucki G. International classification of functioning, disability, and health (ICF): a promising framework and classification for rehabilitation medicine. Am J Phys Med Rehabil 2005;84:733–40.
3. Simons M. The ICF: foundations for a common understanding of measurement. Burns 2004;30:409–10.
4. Falder S, Browne A, Edgar D, et al. Core outcome measures for adult burn survivors: a clinical overview. Burns 2009;35:618–41.
5. van Baar ME, Essink-Bot ML, Oen IM, et al. Functional outcome after burns: a review. Burns 2006;32:1–9.
6. Brych SB, Engrav LH, Rivara FP, et al. Time off work and return to work rates after burns: systematic review of the literature and a large two-center series. J Burn Care Rehabil 2001;22:401–5.
7. Esselman PC, Wiechman Askay S, Carrougher GJ, et al. Barriers to return to work after burn injuries. Arch Phys Med Rehabil 2007;88(Suppl 2):S50–6.

8. Schneider JC, Bassi S, Ryan CM. Barriers impacting employment after burn injury. J Burn Care Res 2009;30:294–300.

9. Hwang YF, Chen-Sea MJ, Chen CL. Factors related to return to work and job modifications after a hand burn. J Burn Care Res 2009;30:661–7.

10. Chapman TT, Richard RL, Hedman TL, et al. Military return to duty and civilian return to work factors following buns with focus on the hand and literature review. J Burn Care Res 2008;29:756–62.

11. Fauerbach JA, Engrav L, Kowalske K, et al. Barriers to employment among working-aged patients with major burn injury. J Burn Care Rehabil 2001;22: 26–34.

12. Quinn T, Wasiak J, Cleland H. An examination of factors that affect return to work following burns: a systematic review of the literature. Burns 2010;36(7):1021–6.

13. Wrigley M, Trotman K, Dimick A, et al. Factors relating to return to work after burn injury. J Burn Care Rehabil 1995;16:445–50.

14. Dyster-Aas J, Kildal M, Willebrand M, et al. Work status and burn specific health after work-related burn injury. Burns 2004;30:839–42.

15. Dyster-Aas J, Kildal M, Willebrand M. Return to work and health-related quality of life after burn injury. J Rehabil Med 2007;39:49–55.

16. Öster C, Kildal M, Ekselius L. Return to work after burn injury: burn-injured individuals' perception of barriers and facilitators. J Burn Care Res 2010;31:540–50.

17. Mackey SP, Diba R, McKeown D, et al. Return to work after burns: a qualitative research study. Burns 2009;35:338–42.

18. Noble J, Gomez M, Fish JS. Quality of life and return to work following electrical burns. Burns 2006;32:159–64.

19. Theman K, Singerman J, Gomez M, et al. Return to work after low voltage electrical injuries. J Burn Care Res 2008;29:959–64.

20. Chudasama S, Goverman J, Donaldson JH, et al. Does voltage predict return to work and neuropsychiatric sequelae following electrical burn injury? Ann Plast Surg 2010;64:522–5.

21. Staley M, Anderson L, Greenhalgh D, et al. Return to school as an outcome measure after a burn injury. J Burn Care Rehabil 1999;20:91–4.

22. Christiansen M, Carrougher GJ, Engrav LH, et al. Time to school re-entry after burn injury is quite short. J Burn Care Res 2007;28:478–81.

23. Blakeney P, Moore P, Meyer W, et al. Efficacy of school reentry programs. J Burn Care Rehabil 1995;16:469–72.

24. The journey back: resources to assist school reentry after burn injury. Grand Rapids (MI): Phoenix Society for Burn Survivors; 2006.

Index

Note: Page numbers of article titles are in **boldface** type.

A

Age, as factor in burn injuries, 202
Alopecia, burn-related, procedures for, 319
Amputation(s), burn-related, electrical burns, 270
Amputation, burn-related, prosthetic after, **277–299**. See also *Burn amputation, prosthetic after.*
Analgesia/analgesics, hypnotic, in burn injury–related pain management, 334
Antimicrobial agents, topical, for burn injuries, 208–211
Arthritis, septic, burn injury–related, 267–268
Axilla, burn injuries of, reconstruction of, 323

B

Biologic dressings, in burn wound care, 210–211, 218
Biopsychosocial model of recovery, for burn injuries, 327–331
Body image, dissatisfaction with, as factor in psychosocial recovery after burn injuries, 339–340
Bone(s), exposed, in burn wound care, 222
Bone metabolism, burn injury effects on, 265–266
Bony changes, electrical burn injury–related, 270
Breast reconstruction, burn injury–related, 322
Burn alopecia, procedures for, 319
Burn amputation
   described, 277
   patient goals after, 279–282
     desensitization, 279–280
     education, 280
     family and peer influences on, 280–282
     medical justification in, 282
     setting of, 280
   pre-prosthetic evaluation and training after, 278–279
     electrical vs. thermal mechanisms in, 278
     ROM limitations in, 279
     sensation compromise in, 279
   prosthetic after
     description of, 282–283
     management of, **277–299**
     prescription for lower extremity, 283–288
       alignment, 288
       foot/ankle, 288
       interface, 284–285
       knee, 286

Phys Med Rehabil Clin N Am 22 (2011) 357–365
doi:10.1016/S1047-9651(11)00053-2
1047-9651/11/$ – see front matter © 2011 Elsevier Inc. All rights reserved.
pmr.theclinics.com

Moving?

Make sure your subscription moves with you!

To notify us of your new address, find your **Clinics Account Number** (located on your mailing label above your name), and contact customer service at:

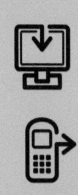

Email: journalscustomerservice-usa@elsevier.com

800-654-2452 (subscribers in the U.S. & Canada)
314-447-8871 (subscribers outside of the U.S. & Canada)

Fax number: 314-447-8029

Elsevier Health Sciences Division
Subscription Customer Service
3251 Riverport Lane
Maryland Heights, MO 63043

*To ensure uninterrupted delivery of your subscription, please notify us at least 4 weeks in advance of move.

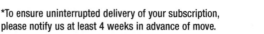

Printed and bound by CPI Group (UK) Ltd, Croydon, CR0 4YY

03/10/2024

01040444-0011